"*A Radical Guide for Women with ADHD* is more than a workbook only for women with attention deficit/hyperactivity disorder (ADHD). It is a beautifully written, inspiring resource and tool that every human being living with shame, blame, and misperceived negative emotions of being 'less than' needs to refer to daily. Sari Solden and Michelle Frank have created a transformational guide with exercises, questions, and inspiring stories that will immediately encourage readers to explore and discover their inner greatness. I highly recommend this workbook for coaches, therapists, physicians, and every human being who truly wants to discover the true essence of who they are and want to be in the world."

> —**David Giwerc, MCC, MCAC**, founder and president, ADD Coach Academy; master certified ADHD coach, PAAC; master certified coach, ICF; and author of *Permission to Proceed*

"In this easy-to-read workbook, Sari Solden and Michelle Frank invite women with ADHD to recognize and challenge a variety of assumptions about themselves and others that may needlessly prevent them from experiencing their own full potential. The authors use brief examples from women of various ages to show that constructive, positive change is quite possible with ADHD. Many women with ADHD will find this book interesting, challenging, and helpful."

> —**Thomas E. Brown, PhD**, director, Brown Clinic for Attention and Related Disorders, Manhattan Beach, CA; adjunct clinical associate professor in the department of psychiatry, Keck School of Medicine of USC; and author of *Smart But Stuck* and *Outside the Box*

"To say this is *the* book about and for women with ADHD is only part of the story. This is a book that warmly promotes self-compassion and the true soul work that is essential for living a valued, successful life with ADHD. Be prepared to see yourself in these pages. You will engage in hearty laughter and cry tears of validation and forgiveness. Most of all, you won't feel alone as you will feel completely understood by the authors."

> —**Roberto Olivardia, PhD**, clinical psychologist, and lecturer in the department of psychiatry at Harvard Medical School

"I was in tears when I began reading this book. Even though I'm many years into my own ADHD journey—and, I thought (wrongly), past the feelings of anger, sadness, and loss—the memories of that early pain of hiding, shame, and negative self-talk returned in a flash as I read vignettes of the authors' clients as well as their own personal stories. This is a book about courage. Solden and Frank embrace you—the reader—and travel along with you, sharing new ways to see yourself, not just as a woman with ADHD, but as a woman with so much to offer. ADHD may be an invisible condition, but it doesn't mean you have to be invisible in order to feel safe from criticism—internal or external. You don't need to hide anymore. And that is such a relief. This book is now on the top of my must-read list that I share with all of my clients."

—**Terry Matlen, LMSW, ACSW**, psychotherapist, author of *The Queen of Distraction*, and founder of www.addconsults.com

"Sari Solden, for years the great pioneer in working with women and ADHD, has now teamed up with Michelle Frank to create this dynamic, valuable workbook that will help women embolden themselves to break out of whatever self-imposed exiles they may have lived in and soar to the heights they deserve and will love."

—**Edward Hallowell, MD**, coauthor of *Driven to Distraction*

"In this marvelous workbook, Sari Solden and Michelle Frank sensitively guide women with ADHD to increase their understanding and self-acceptance; stop feeling shame, hiding, and listening to negative messages; identify and pursue their special talents and dreams; restore wholeness and authenticity; connect meaningfully with others; use professional help wisely; and create an effective action plan for living fully as women with ADHD in an empowered way. Above all, from the first to the last word, the authors show a level of understanding and empathy for women with ADHD, along with an ability to help them, that goes light years beyond all similar books."

—**Arthur L. Robin, PhD**, licensed clinical psychologist, and coauthor of *Adult ADHD-Focused Couple Therapy*

"Finally! An ADHD-friendly guidebook that skirts the dizzying array of superficial strategies to address the powerful inner lives of ADHD women. Its write-in-the-book format creates a journal that is deeply personal and potentially life-changing. Poignant, yet practical, *A Radical Guide for Women with ADHD* is a beacon call for authenticity—a bedrock for every ADHD woman. Destined to be a classic must-read: Five++ stars!"

—**Linda Roggli, PCC**, ADDiva Network for ADHD Women 40-and-better,
author of *Confessions of an ADDiva*, and cofounder of ADHD Women's Palooza

"Instead of offering the usual fixes or treatments for ADHD, this truly radical book shows women with ADHD how to live an authentic life, one free from stigma and shame. With helpful worksheets and practical, inspirational prose, this is a must-read for women with ADHD and the clinicians who work with them."

—**Susan Caughman**, editor-in-chief, *ADDitude* magazine

"You can only begin to believe in yourself when someone believes in you. Sari and Michelle offer that belief. Their faith in the potential and power of women with ADHD is refreshing. It takes bravery to stop hiding. Buying this book is an act of bravery. It's the first step to believing in yourself. To believing you are capable of much more than camouflaging yourself as normal.

This is not a book of strategies to help you appear normal. This is a guide to help you do the important work that comes before ADHD strategies can be effective. Don't misunderstand—strategies are essential when you live with ADHD. But are you looking for strategies that will allow you to reach your goals? Or are you looking for strategies that will help you blend in with the neurotypicals? Without understanding, you cannot accept. Without acceptance, there is no path to living out loud with ADHD.

As I read, I found myself enjoying the interactivity. Sari and Michelle have a warm, conversational tone. They share ideas in an always caring and sometimes humorous way. They include stories from other women with ADHD, reaffirming you are not alone. And throughout, they ask you questions that encourage you to get to know yourself better. No one has all the answers. They sure don't have YOUR answers! Sari and Michelle never pretend they have all the answers. I love that they help you ask the right questions. I wish I had this book twenty years ago. Save yourself twenty years; get it today."

—**Duane Gordon**, president of the Attention Deficit Disorder Association (ADDA)

"Sari and Michelle are your super-smart, empathic friends who have been there before you and want to save you a lot of unnecessary suffering. They won't tell you what to do, but, like any good friends, they will help you figure out what you want to do. Your ADHD symptoms may or may not be better after reading this wise, insightful book, but your life definitely will be."

—**Ari Tuckman, PsyD, CST**, author of *ADHD After Dark*

"Congratulations, Sari and Michelle, for writing a wonderful guide for helping women with ADHD learn to legitimize rather than stigmatize human differences. Your insights support and also add to our lessons learned from resilient individuals who lead meaningful and productive lives in the face of adversity and challenge. You did an excellent job as well in reminding us of the important role that human understanding can play in rising above a difficult past, and the role that human misunderstanding can play in prolonging one. A countless number of women with ADHD will grow stronger and more resilient as a result of your new book."

—**Mark Katz, PhD**, clinical and consulting psychologist in San Diego, CA, and author of *Children Who Fail at School But Succeed at Life* and *On Playing a Poor Hand Well*

"Whether newly diagnosed or dealing with her challenges for decades, there is something for every woman living with ADHD in *A Radical Guide for Women with ADHD*. Michelle and Sari's deep understanding and authentic, sometimes painful accounts of living with ADHD are evidence of their own experience and expertise, and give a sense of encouragement and reassurance for the reader. The reflection and discovery exercises offer an opportunity to learn about ourselves, celebrate our strengths, and indeed become our bravest, brightest, and boldest selves. This book is the new must-read for every woman of any age with ADHD."

—**Evelyn Polk Green, MEd, MSEd**, ADHD advocate; past president of the Attention Deficit Disorder Association (ADDA) and Children and Adults with ADHD (CHADD)

"Sari Solden literally wrote the first major book on women and ADHD, and in this 2019 presentation with Michelle Frank, brings it all up to date. Whether you're a woman with ADHD, or a friend, intimate, or family member, you'll find both revelation and reassurance within these pages."

—**Thom Hartmann**, author of *Attention Deficit Disorder* and *Adult ADHD*

A RADICAL GUIDE FOR

Women with ADHD

Embrace Neurodiversity,
Live Boldly, *and*
Break Through Barriers

SARI SOLDEN, MS

MICHELLE FRANK, PsyD

New Harbinger Publications, Inc.

Publisher's Note

This publication is designed to provide accurate and authoritative information in regard to the subject matter covered. It is sold with the understanding that the publisher is not engaged in rendering psychological, financial, legal, or other professional services. If expert assistance or counseling is needed, the services of a competent professional should be sought.

Distributed in Canada by Raincoast Books

Copyright © 2019 by Sari Solden and Michelle Frank
           New Harbinger Publications, Inc.
           5674 Shattuck Avenue
           Oakland, CA 94609
           www.newharbinger.com

Cover design by Amy Shoup

Acquired by Elizabeth Hollis Hansen

Edited by Marisa Solis

All Rights Reserved

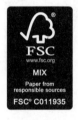 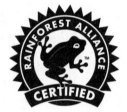

Library of Congress Cataloging-in-Publication Data on file

Book printed in the United States of America

23   22   21

10   9   8   7   6   5

We dedicate this book to our clients, who give us the privilege of sharing their stories and dreams, and who inspire us every day. So much of what we know about how to live brave, bright, and bold lives as women with ADHD comes from them.

Contents

PART III: **Bolder**

Foreword

In 1995, I was waiting in line to attend a talk at a conference organized by Children and Adults with Attention Deficit/Hyperactivity Disorder (CHADD). I noticed that the woman in front of me held a book titled *Women with Attention Deficit Disorder*. At a time when the neuropsychiatric community regularly rejected that girls were capable of being diagnosed with ADHD, let alone women, I couldn't believe my good fortune. I said to her, "Whoever wrote that book is a genius!" and she replied, "I wrote it." That was my introduction to Sari Solden.

Historically, ADHD described the unmanageable behavior of hyperactive young boys. Because most females did not display these behaviors, they didn't meet the male-based criteria for diagnosis. In fact, at that very conference, a keynote speaker dismissively termed these girls and women "ADD wannabes."

ADHD women were living like refugees: First, they were marginalized because they didn't conform to society's gender role expectations of empathy, organization, and compliance. Second, they were marginalized because they didn't meet the criteria laid out in the *Diagnostic and Statistical Manual of Mental Disorders*. Too different to measure on society's yardstick, but not different enough to be permitted the relief of a neurological explanation, women with ADHD were left to attribute their differences to their worst fears. Invalidated and misunderstood, many internalized the harshest criticisms.

From our current vantage point, we can see that Solden's bold and honest words changed the landscape of ADHD forever. I do not believe it to be an overstatement to say that she unlocked the psychic prison isolating women with ADHD. We know this to be true because the response was thunderous; women around the world felt empowered by the simple knowledge that they were not alone, and that their struggle had a name. Now, Sari Solden and coauthor Michelle Frank propel the conversation forward once again. Their book encourages women to claim their space in the world and make themselves seen, heard, and known.

It is both unsettling and ironic that the radical idea that this book promotes is self-acceptance. Despite the ever-changing zeitgeist, women strive to conform if they can; women with ADHD implore clinicians to "make me normal."

For those with low self-esteem, an all-too-common coping mechanism is the construction of a false self. This is a devastating dynamic in which some individuals are not afforded the empathy and validation that most enjoy. After repeated rejections, they conclude that they are not the kind valued by society. A desperate solution ensues: designing a false self that mimics neurotypicals and that may allow them to pass for "normal."

At first consideration, it may seem a brilliant disguise. But Solden and Frank make clear that when women with ADHD compensate for their challenges, it comes at a high emotional cost: hypervigilant and depleted, they are still haunted by stigma and shame. When women with ADHD appear to not have any symptoms when out in the world, they may celebrate it as a success. Ironically, the result of coping well is that their plight remains secret yet no less damaging. Rather than solicit support, they dread the inevitable crack in the facade that may expose them as an impostor. In fact, as Leonard Cohen wrote, "There is a crack in everything; that's how the light gets in." And so, those cracks in the facade don't need to be fixed—those slices of light illuminate their radiant true selves.

If you are among thousands of women who have been shamed, discredited, and silenced, allow Sari Solden and Michelle Frank to be your fierce yet compassionate guides. They understand that, after decades of hiding, fears can paralyze. Your authors patiently nurture resilience and courage. They offer the opportunity to understand your role in the world by seeing it from a position of acceptance and compassion. Brimming with empathy, they offer an oasis where it is safe for women to begin the process of untangling their self-worth from their brain wiring. In this breathtakingly diverse world of ours, Solden and Frank's *A Radical Guide for Women with ADHD* dares to celebrate all these fascinating and unique individuals.

—Ellen B. Littman, PhD

Clinical psychologist in independent practice in New York
Coauthor of *Understanding Girls with ADHD*

A Note to Our Readers

We are delighted to serve as your guides on this exciting journey on which you are about to embark. Here are a few important, brief clarifications of some of the terms and concepts used in this book.

Enjoy the ride!

Some ADHD Basics, Because It Gets Confusing!

This workbook is intended for women who have attention deficit/hyperactivity disorder (ADHD) and those who help them and love them. Because we can't include everything we know about ADHD, this book assumes some familiarity with most ADHD basics. To help you follow along with our discussion of certain aspects of ADHD throughout this book, however, we want to explain a few essential bits of background information, including what we mean when we talk about ADHD and its various presentations. While we most commonly use the general term "ADHD" in this book, at times, when important, we specify a type of presentation.

Yes, They're Calling It ADHD These Days

There is a lot of confusion around the name and signifiers of the diagnosis of ADHD, because the diagnostic label itself has changed several times during the course of many decades. Today, the current correct diagnostic terminology is *attention deficit/hyperactivity disorder,* or ADHD, which is further delineated by the diagnostic manual into three subtypes: predominantly inattentive presentation, predominantly hyperactive/impulsive presentation, and combined presentation.

Sometimes you will hear the names "ADHD" and "ADD" used interchangeably. This is because attention deficit disorder, or ADD, was the prior diagnostic term used in the 1980 edition of the diagnostic manual, and people simply got used to the name. Though occasionally people still casually use the term ADD to indicate ADHD without hyperactivity, or the predominantly inattentive presentation, this terminology is outdated and incorrect.

Predominantly Inattentive Presentation. People who have the predominantly inattentive presentation of ADHD present primarily with great difficulty getting going or activating to do things (even when they want or need to), disorganization, forgetfulness, distractibility, zoning out, misperception of time, and emotional dysregulation. They don't struggle with hyperactivity and impulsivity as much as those who have other subtypes of the condition. Instead, some tend to be underactive instead of hyperactive.

Predominantly Hyperactive/Impulsive Presentation. People who have the predominantly hyperactive/impulsive presentation of ADHD struggle a great deal with hyperactivity. They too struggle with inattentive traits, but their main challenges are related to hyperarousal and trouble "putting on the brakes." People with this subtype have difficulty sitting still, waiting in line, and holding back impulses to act and speak. They are fidgety and feel a constant need to be "on the go" or have an inner sense of restlessness. They also struggle with impulsivity and tend to have experienced a lot of negative consequences from uninhibited behaviors, hasty comments, and rash decision-making. Men are more likely to be diagnosed with the predominantly hyperactive/impulsive presentation.

Combined Presentation. People with the combined presentation of ADHD have aspects of both the inattentive and hyperactive/impulsive presentations. Women with combined presentation often describe experiences similar to those with the inattentive presentation, along with being overly talkative, prone to interrupting conversations, making impulsive decisions, and physical or mental hyperactivity.

ADHD and Executive Functioning

What most people know about ADHD is only a small pixel of the big picture. ADHD isn't necessarily a deficit of attention so much as a problem regulating various aspects of cognition, emotion, and behavior. It also doesn't necessarily mean someone is hyper. So what is it?

ADHD is a lifelong, neurobehavioral, genetic syndrome that leads to structural, chemical, communication, and arousal differences in the brain that subsequently impact what is called the "executive functioning" system of the brain.

Dr. Thomas Brown aptly describes ADHD as:

> a complex syndrome of developmental impairments of executive function, the self-management system of the brain, a system of mostly unconscious operations. These impairments are situationally variable, chronic and significantly interfere with functioning in many aspects of the person's daily life. (2013, 20)

The operations that Brown refers to are called *executive functioning skills*, which he groups into several clusters, including: activation and initiation of tasks, focus and sustained attention, regulation of alertness, effort and processing speed, emotional regulation, working memory abilities, and self-regulation of behaviors. Brown provides an excellent description of these clusters and what they mean for day-to-day life with ADHD in several of his books and articles, some of which are cited at the end of this book, including *A New Understanding of ADHD in Children and Adults*. We hope you look over his work, if you haven't already done so; it is sure to be validating and enlightening!

In the pages that follow, you will hear us refer to the challenges of ADHD as often originating from a dysregulation of the executive functioning system and related skills. While an in-depth description of these terms is out of the scope of this project, we want you to understand that challenges with these management functions of the brain cause many of the struggles for women and are very descriptive of the way you may experience ADHD.

What If I Haven't Been Diagnosed with ADHD but I Think I Have It?

If you suspect you have ADHD, it is important to meet with a professional who has some experience in diagnosing and treating the condition. There is a free checklist that screens for the presence of common symptoms of ADHD at http://www.add.org that you can complete and take with you to your first visit. A psychiatrist, physician, psychologist, clinical social worker, or therapist can diagnose ADHD. Ask potential providers if they have worked with women with ADHD, have attended any trainings or conferences on ADHD in recent years, and are familiar with ADHD as an executive functioning dysregulation.

Am I Doomed?

Nope! ADHD is a brain-based difference that doesn't go away, but it is not a death sentence. You can—and will—live a happy, healthy, fulfilling life as a woman with ADHD, we promise. We've got your back and some ideas that we think will help, so keep reading!

Composite Characters

The stories in this book are composite depictions of a large group of women we have known and with whom we have worked throughout the years. We share these stories in the hopes that you may find commonalities in the experiences of other women at every stage of the journey. All of the names used are fictional, and the details of any particular woman's story has been greatly altered and combined with other similar stories in order to protect confidentiality.

PART I

Braver

"And the day came when the risk to remain tight in a bud was more painful than the risk it took to blossom."

—Anaïs Nin

You probably understand what we mean when we say that having ADHD can feel like you have something wonderful inside, just waiting to bloom, if only you could break free from all of the things holding you back. You might have found yourself hiding away more and more as you've tried your very best to manage your challenges and cope with the hurt, loss, and confusion that comes with ADHD life. You may have tried, time and again, to fix yourself, hoping to find freedom in becoming more like someone else, someone without ADHD, only to discover that you can't get rid of the hard stuff without also getting rid of the splendor that makes you who you are or without living behind a tiring facade.

If you picked up this book, chances are you're ready to drop the old struggle and put your energy into something new and bold. Because, as you've likely found, there comes a time when sacrificing who you are—who you know yourself to be and what you most deeply long to become—is more painful than facing the fear of opening up to be seen, heard, and known for all that you are. So stop waiting—this moment is as good as any. It is time to take the risk to blossom. So let's begin…bravely!

CHAPTER 1

Welcome to the Tribe
Making a World of Difference

Our book is called a "radical" guide for women with ADHD to emphasize the simple but "radical" idea that instead of trying to change and *fix* herself, a woman with ADHD can simply learn to *be* herself. This guide is not radical in the sense of promoting any unusual strategies, herbs, or diets, or discarding effective, conventional treatment for the brain-based challenges of ADHD. To be clear, this book is not anti-medication or anti-strategy.

This book is about ADHD. But, the truth is, it's not entirely or exclusively about ADHD. It's about a great deal more. At its core, this guidebook is about helping you become and value who you truly are—challenges and all. For this reason, our approach places an emphasis on embracing brain differences and recognizing that the process of helping women with ADHD is incredibly nuanced and complex.

The ways in which people with brain-based differences are pathologized and compared is similar to how others with more visible differences are judged by a gold standard of the majority. With the concept of *neurodiversity*, Thomas Armstrong (2010) addresses the much healthier and broader way of celebrating and understanding those with brain-based differences instead of viewing them as inferior. "Instead of pretending there is hidden away in a vault somewhere a perfectly 'normal' brain to which all other brains must be compared, we need to admit there is no standard brain, just as there is no standard flower, or standard cultural or racial group, and that in fact diversity among brains is just as wonderfully enriching as biodiversity and the diversity among cultures and races" (2–3).

To help our clients with these unique brain-based challenges come to embrace their neuro-diversity, we guide them through a process of *untangling* in which they come to terms with who they are at their core—under all those layers of shame, stigma, and confusion. We have watched the exciting process that unfolds as women with ADHD eventually break through cultural, internal, and relational barriers to move beyond surviving to actually leading bold lives as powerful and strong women with unique brains, strengths, and challenges.

Better Together

You are not an alien on this planet or a stranger in this life of yours. You are part of a community of extraordinary women, kindred companions on the journey through an ADHD life that is full of more wonder and chaos than you think you can handle. (You can handle it, by the way—you already are!) And in this community you will find solace in the stories of one another.

We are psychotherapists in our professional lives, but we are also women on the same journey as you. Over the years, we have had the privilege and pleasure of accompanying and guiding women from all over the world on this exciting journey of discovery. Remember that you are not alone on this wild ride.

It takes courage to keep going when you aren't completely sure where you are supposed to be headed. (We've been there too.) Uncertain as you might feel, at some point you need to embrace your differences and difficulties, and move on to own your gifts, talents, and the qualities that make you who you are. You will have to work at this, fight for it.

For women with the kinds of mysterious and invisible differences that come with ADHD, it takes a special kind of courage to keep the spark alive and to keep opening, slowly but surely, until we blossom, no longer hiding who we are.

At some point, ADHD has probably impacted your ability to let yourself be known, to say what you think, or show who you are. The truth is, this journey to living boldly as a woman with ADHD isn't completely about ADHD. It is also about how you view and express your true self as a woman with invisible differences, which are challenges that other people can't see from the outside.

The way you think about yourself and your ADHD challenges is deeply sculpted by the gradual and eventual internalization of repeated messages about difference, the implied consequences of living outside the majority—*neurotypical** and otherwise—and how those belief systems continue to shape your internal and external experiences in the present. It's important to

---

*   "Neurotypical" is a term that has become increasingly popular in clinical and scholastic settings to describe individuals who are considered neurologically "typical," or without differences such as ADHD, an autism spectrum condition, a learning disability, or other similar neurological or neurodevelopmental challenge. Conversely, individuals with ADHD would be considered *neuro-atypical* or *neuro-divergent*. These terms are not absolute medical or psychological descriptors and do not hold any sort of judgment or assertion as to the "right" way to be in the world; they simply help differentiate between those who fall within the average range of functioning on most things and those who demonstrate more variable brain-based challenges.

understand your relationship to the idea of *difference*, because this is exactly the world us women with ADHD inhabit: a world of difference.

Redefining ADHD Treatment

The complexity of ADHD treatment is this: it isn't until you are able to fully identify, accept, and respect your differences that you are truly able to fully engage in the change process. Until then, you will find yourself fighting an uphill, unwinnable battle against yourself. In the words of another psychotherapist: "The curious paradox is that when I accept myself just as I am, then I change" (Rogers 1961, 17).

ADHD has consistently been shown to be a genetic, chronic, brain-based condition that involves structural, chemical, and communication differences that subsequently impact cognition, emotion, and behavior, specifically those related to what are known as the *executive functions* of the brain.

Thomas E. Brown (2005) uses the metaphor of a symphony orchestra to describe the executive functioning system of the brain as a manager of cognitive functions.

> Imagine a symphony orchestra in which each musician plays his or her instrument very well. If there is no conductor to organize the orchestra and start the players together, to signal the introduction of the woodwinds or the fading out of the strings, or to convey an overall interpretation of the music to all players, the orchestra will not produce good music. Symptoms of ADHD can be compared to impairments not in the individual musicians, but in the orchestra's conductor. (10)

These management functions of the brain can affect your ability to activate yourself enough to begin a task, to sustain focus once you start the task, and to stick with it when your energy or interest wanes—and that's just for starters! For more on understanding executive functioning we direct you to our comprehensive list of resources at the website for this book: http://www.newharbinger.com/32617 (see the very back of this book for instructions on how to access this site).

Understanding executive functioning helps us begin to see how, for women, challenges with organizing, coordinating, prioritizing, maintaining routines, managing time, and remembering details can collide with our internalized "job description" and play havoc with the way we feel about ourselves and our challenges (Solden 2005, 58–59).

The True "Radical" Goal of Treatment

Consider for a moment how you have been thinking about your ADHD and what you have been told or come to believe about ADHD treatment goals.

What if we asked you to consider a change in the way you thought about treatment for ADHD? What if a shift in how you describe your treatment goals and how you relate to yourself as a woman with ADHD was the missing key to making treatment really, truly work? Would you be willing to try that?

We believe that the goal of ADHD treatment should not be to get over, fundamentally change, or otherwise contort who you are, but to move toward your hopes and dreams, to deepen your relationship with your authentic self, and to use your strengths and voice to create spaces and relationships that work for you.

What if the goal of treatment is to make it easier to access more of who you truly are, not to get over who you are?

We ask you to consider accepting yourself and your challenges. Not to become resigned, not to be passive, but to begin a process of real and satisfying change in your life toward meaning and connection.

We absolutely recommend all the effective strategies out there for addressing your ADHD challenges. We just don't want you to wait until you are perfectly organized before you let yourself have a life! Medication, therapy, coaching, and other ADHD-friendly interventions will make it much easier to be *more* of who you really are—not less. This is the true goal of any treatment. Strategies and organizational help should make life easier for you and calm your inner distress, but they should not be approached as a way to fix "damaged goods" or turn you into someone other than yourself.

We know, without a doubt, that tackling the issue of shame is absolutely imperative for people with ADHD. In fact, many renowned ADHD professionals and researchers have begun to emphasize the importance of this deeper work as an essential element of ADHD treatment (Hinshaw 2018; Hallowell and Dodson 2018). This book will take you on a journey that embraces this groundbreaking evolution in ADHD treatment.

> *What if the goal of treatment is to make it easier to access more of who you truly are, not to get over who you are?*

Until you feel comfortable with the idea of differences, you will spend your life with ADHD pretending, placating, hiding, and feeling ashamed. It can take a long time to get to a place where you can make a shift in your ideas about ADHD, depending on your early life experiences. Just remember: it doesn't matter what medication you take or what shiny new organizational system you try: you won't get there as long as your goal is to get over who you are.

What follows is the first of many Reflection questions that you will encounter throughout this workbook. You may want to get a journal if you find that you need more room to write and develop your ideas.

Reflection: Treatment Goals

What immediately comes to mind when you think of ADHD treatment?

_____

_____

Consider what it would look like if some of your goals included:

- Moving toward my hopes and dreams

- Deepening my relationship with myself

- Using my strengths

- Using my voice

- Creating spaces that work better for me

- Building mutual and satisfying relationships

- Finding it easier to access more of who I truly am

Only Dogs and Furniture Need Fixing

Many women with ADHD have a deeply ingrained hope that a few sessions of ADHD-oriented therapy will "fix" them. The sooner, the better!

We live in a quick-fix culture. Sitting with the uncertainty of a slowly unfolding process is not easy for anyone and palatable to few. The reality of the situation, however, is that you are not a problem to be solved.

We offer no quick, absolute solution, because even within moments of ADHD hardships, we see opportunity, not deficit. Rest assured, it is okay to have these thoughts, fears, and questions. You don't have to view ADHD as a "gift" in order to move forward. It may take a while for you to feel comfortable internalizing the idea that you don't need fixing. And you may be concerned that we, the authors, are invalidating the struggles inherent in living with ADHD. We are not.

We, as clinicians and as women with ADHD, absolutely know the struggle. And we have found that colluding with the desire to fundamentally fix yourself, your life, and your brain is incredibly harmful to the process of ultimately finding the peace and joy you most desire. In fact, the goal of "repair and replace" can completely sabotage your attempts to better manage your ADHD symptoms. So though it may initially make you feel a bit uncomfortable, trust us when we say that trying to fix yourself never works. Consider that you could stop trying so hard and drop the struggle. (We promise it isn't going anywhere and you won't miss it!) What's stopping you? You don't have much to lose, aside from shame, doubt, and self-deprecation!

Now we come to the first of many Discovery exercises, which provide examples of experiences common to women with ADHD. Many of these exercises include prompts or suggestions to get your wheels turning; some are even accompanied by Reflection exercises that ask you to expand upon your thinking even further. Feel free to jot down any thoughts or feelings that come up.

Discovery: Are We There Yet?

Some versions of the following questions are commonly asked of therapists by women with ADHD. Do you relate to any of these? If so, check off the ones that resonate with you and notice your reactions.

☐ "How bad is it, Doc?"

☐ "Can you help me learn strategies to make me like other women?"

☐ "How many sessions do I need to get over this?"

☐ "Is this going to help me get more organized/be more productive/be less forgetful?"

☐ "How do I get over this case of terminal uniqueness?"

What's So Bad About Being Different Anyway?

Before we go deeper, it's important to know what you have internalized about the meaning of *difference*.

Many of the messages and limiting beliefs that we as women with ADHD have deeply internalized come from our early experiences with differences and the perceptions of those close to us. Oftentimes, these messages contribute greatly to the tangles that keep us trapped in layers of shame, guilt, fear, and general not-good-enough-ness. To explore these tangles, we have to be aware of what happens within systems (relationships, communities, groups, etc.) when one person or a group of people dares to be different or to reveal their differences.

🪷 *Kim's Story:* Differences Disrupt the Family

When Kim struggled with traditional schooling, her parents, who wanted her to follow in their footsteps and become a physician, told her, "You just need to apply yourself and try harder." When she expressed interest in majoring in history, her parents commented, "Don't be ridiculous," as they rolled their eyes and walked away. For Kim, expressing difference was interpreted as strange, threatening, and unacceptable. Those "small" messages have a lot of power.

For many of us, expression of difference has, at least at some point, led to obstacles. As a rule, systems of all kinds resist change, because the group members are familiar and comfortable with the "way things have always been"—even if that way has always been unhealthy. Resistance to change and divergence acts as a type of unconscious group survival mechanism—helpful or not, fair or not, kind or not.

The goals outlined in this workbook greatly surpass and exceed learning to be organized. This book will help you learn to:

- Separate your core identity from your brain-based challenges

- Stop allowing yourself to be diminished

- Be a whole person who feels complete within your own skin, brain, and life

- Be close to others, while still protecting yourself

- Lean into your ADHD challenges, so that you can manage your symptoms

- Find ways to fill yourself up, instead of giving everything away

In order to move into a place of living comfortably with your ADHD, instead of fighting against it, you have to bring awareness to some deep, perhaps barely noticed beliefs and fears about what it means to be a woman with a different way of being in the world. Let's explore what you learned in your early years about what it means to express differences.

🪷 *Brianna's Story:* Get over Yourself!

Twenty-seven-year-old Brianna recalls many messages and mistreatment related to both the visible and the invisible aspects of her identity as a woman of color who has ADHD. These messages ingrained a sense of separation, a dismissal of her rights and needs, and a silencing of her voice. Even within her family, full of high achievers, Brianna became acutely aware of messages that she should minimize her difficulties and that challenges should be surpassed, not coddled. Her teachers, noting how smart she was, refused to "indulge" her by repeating instructions or granting other reasonable accommodations when she asked for help.

Brianna continues to struggle with the messages she's received her whole life: "Everybody struggles, so deal with it—alone and silently." "Your needs aren't a priority and your voice won't be valued." "What makes you think you get special treatment?"

Discovery: Expressing Differences

Check off any of the adjectives below that complete the sentence in a way that's familiar to you, or add your own.

As a girl, I learned that expressing difference was…

☐ Dangerous

☐ Blasphemous   Or…

☐ Threatening   ☐ Respected

☐ Rude   ☐ Encouraged

☐ Mean   ☐ Creative and independent

☐ Disrespectful   ☐ A good thing

☐ Pointless   ☐ Powerful

☐ Disconnecting   ☐ Essential

☐ Shameful   ☐ Freeing

☐ _____   ☐ _____

Reflection: Expressing Differences

Think back and let yourself remember what you learned about the dangers of expressing differences when you were growing up.

When you think about the concept of difference—whether visible or invisible, your own or that of others—what feelings or thoughts pop up?

_____

_____

_____

_____

Looking back, how were you different from your family in big and small ways?

_____

_____

_____

_____

To what degree were your differences encouraged or tolerated?

_____

_____

_____

_____

What views did you hear expressed about the differences of others—visible or invisible—in your family, community, or in the general culture?

_____

_____

_____

_____

Were you encouraged to speak your own mind, or was it threatening to stand out? What impact did that have on you? How might it continue to affect you?

_____

_____

_____

_____

Where Ideas About Difference Come From

Nothing is wrong with difference; it's a beautiful thing. However, difference can also be threatening to tightly woven webs of social patterns, roles, and hierarchies of power. When group norms promote fear of differences, these beliefs flow through generations, communities, and families insidiously. It takes a great deal of awareness, introspection, courage, and assertiveness to break free from these invisible chains of fear.

We are all inextricably linked to our social, historical, and family contexts. If you look back on a message you received from your mother, for instance, you may be able to quickly identify where she got the idea from in the first place. Perhaps from her own mother, who in turn got those ideas from her family's experiences of racial discrimination, economic privilege or scarcity, religious persecution, the shadow of family secrets, the trauma of generations of alcoholism, or simply trying to keep up with the Joneses.

Reflection: Generational Experiences

Did a few thoughts about your own family history come to mind? Briefly take note of them here.

_____

_____

_____

_____

Social expectations are passed down systemically and multigenerationally within cultures, communities, and families, and are reinforced by public policies and institutions. Even if some of them now seem ridiculous to us when viewed objectively, we can begin to understand why a particular set of norms originated. We can also start to see how powerfully they may continue to operate and impact how we view ourselves in light of our differences and difficulties. In the case of Brianna, understanding how her "go it alone, try harder" mentality developed helped her begin to notice when she was burning out and needing to ask for help.

Accepting ADHD

You likely heard talk of "coming to terms" with ADHD after you received a diagnosis. You might be familiar, either through reading or lived experience, with the "grief cycle" that describes the common stages people go through when coming to terms with life-altering situations (Kübler-Ross 1969). The grief process of denial, anger, bargaining, depression, and acceptance is certainly pertinent to the post-diagnosis journey of adults with ADHD (Solden 2005).

In practice, however, we've noticed that the word "acceptance" is often dismissed, and so the stage that goes with it seems to come in and out of focus, instead of being centering, for women struggling to get to the integration they dream of.

The word "acceptance" seems to be loaded. On the one hand, the word can be used too lightly, as in "Just get on with it already." On the other hand, the actual process of acceptance can be discarded too quickly, as in "Don't resign yourself, try harder."

So, we have a question for you: Have you been resisting the acceptance process when it comes to living with ADHD?

Do you still cling to the narrative of "I just need to try harder. How can I possibly accept this *thing* that makes life so difficult?" We want you to consider that the try-harder mentality is counterproductive. ADHD is a part of you. You were born with it and you will die with it. How has despising and fighting it worked for you so far? How much of your life do you want to spend struggling with, even hating, part of yourself? What has that fixed mind-set truly done for you? Has it moved you closer to where you want to be?

Discovery: **Your Attitudes on Acceptance**

Before moving into acceptance, it is helpful to examine your own attitudes about the process. Do you think that acceptance means any of the following? Check those that apply.

☐ Resignation

☐ Weakness

☐ Giving up

☐ Being passive

☐ Accepting failure

☐ Aiming lower

☐ Other: _____

Fighting against a part of your experience is like trying to punch your way out of quicksand. The more you fight, the more doomed you are to sinking. Dropping the struggle against what distresses you, and thereby moving into acceptance, produces more effective, lasting results than trying to get rid of the distress. The more we avoid that which brings discomfort, the more likely we are to keep having that very discomfort (Hayes, Strosahl, and Wilson 2016).

The concept of acceptance is complex. Beyond the basic level of acceptance, there is something called *radical acceptance*. In her book *Radical Acceptance*, Tara Brach (2003) writes:

Radical acceptance is the necessary antidote to years of neglecting ourselves, years of judging and treating ourselves harshly, years of rejecting this moment's experience. Radical acceptance is the willingness to experience ourselves and our life as it is. (4)

Acceptance is not passive, and it is not resignation; it is an ongoing choice to respect yourself and your circumstance in whatever way it presents in this moment. In fact, you don't have to particularly embrace (or like) your challenges in order to "radically accept" them. From this courageous place of honoring yourself, you can begin to take new actions from a foundation of empowerment and careful discernment of your unique needs and desires.

In short, acceptance is the platform upon which the construction of change is possible. As author Cheryl Strayed (2012, 352) so eloquently put it, "Acceptance is a small, quiet room." It is also the beginning of every meaningful step we take, especially since we all—yes, everyone—will face adversity and struggle at some point in our lives—ADHD or not.

Reflection: Your Attitudes on Acceptance

What does "acceptance" mean to you, especially when thinking about life with ADHD?

_____

_____

What fears come up when you think of acceptance?

_____

_____

What does the "try harder" mentality do for you? What might be some other paths to the same goals or function?

_____

_____

_____

_____

Acceptance means fully knowing who you are—all of who you are—and using that awareness to build a successful and fulfilling life, whatever that may mean for you.

✿ *Paula's Story:* Finding Acceptance

For Paula, acceptance means that, even though she still struggles with organizing her house, her time, and her tasks (despite medication and strategies), she can still direct the focus of her life into her writing, which brings her great peace. She has enjoyed great success and satisfaction by helping the readers of her inspirational blog. Does she still have to deal with the piles of unpaid bills, her messy car, unanswered texts and emails, health insurance claims, belated birthday cards, et cetera? Yes, yes, yes! But she would still have to do all that even if she hadn't made the choice to focus a certain amount of her life pursuing her strength!

Now when Paula returns to the tasks and lists, even though she still experiences ADHD-related stress, she has a much better feeling about herself at the core. These feelings of peace, meaning, purpose, and worth help her see her ADHD challenges in a less judgmental light, and so she is more likely to seek out the unique supports she needs. Paula no longer constantly berates herself for her ADHD challenges, and this makes a huge difference in her well-being and daily functioning.

In summary, the bad news is that you can't "fix" yourself. The good news is there is no need to. (Yes, really.)

ADHD-Friendly Chapter Takeaways

❧ Women with ADHD often harbor shame related to messages they received in child-hood about being a person with differences.

❧ At some point, women with ADHD have to begin the process of accepting their differences.

❧ This is a process that takes work and is more of a gradual unfolding than a sudden decision.

❧ Acceptance does not mean resignation. It means doing away with judgment and moving into a place of self-respect and integration of the reality at hand. This, in turn, frees women with ADHD to approach their lives and their challenges with strength and compassion.

CHAPTER 2

Begin Bravely

Gaining Awareness of How Your Self-Worth Is Tangled Up with Your Challenges

The journey of untangling ADHD from our core identity starts with awareness of our unique life experiences. Becoming aware of how our self-worth has become tangled up with our challenges requires us to take a deep look into our past and our view of ourselves. This takes courage and a leap of faith that what we discover will be beneficial. After all, "Courage is not the absence of fear, but rather the judgment that something else is more important than fear" (Redmoon 1991).

Fear is a hungry beast. It's time to stop feeding it.

Fear is a fierce opponent and competitor for the quality of our life. While we cannot necessarily stop feeling afraid of failure or of being "found out," we can stop giving fear so much power to stop us. We don't win by denying the fear but by refusing to fuel it. Instead, we can make peace with its existence.

One very helpful way to conceptualize this is to think of fear as an annoying passenger on a beautiful cross-county train trip. We can enjoy the picturesque rolling countryside outside the window, the people we meet, and the excitement of traveling to places we have always dreamed of visiting *while also* allowing the annoying, irritating, sometimes intruding other passenger to exist somewhere on the train. Or we can decide: *I'm not going anywhere as long as this annoying person is somewhere on this train with me!* By taking this option, we certainly avoid the unpleasantness (fear), but we will miss the trip altogether (Hayes, Strosahl, and Wilson 2016)! That's because we give the fear the power to take away our joy.

Untangling Your Core from Your Challenges

The hardest part of your journey is dismantling the toxic effect of the insidious, damaging messages of shame and stigma that you, as a woman with invisible differences, have received and internalized during the course of your lifetime. The crux of the ADHD journey has as much to do with letting go of the false beliefs you have about yourself as it does with adding tools and strategies. This is what you need to recognize, first and foremost, because this link—the one that binds your challenges to your worth—is far worse than any symptom of inattention could ever be.

> *The crux of the ADHD journey has as much to do with letting go of the false beliefs you have about yourself as it does with adding tools and strategies.*

Many of us, even those who are quite successful in various ways, still feel constricted by the shame of our unique ADHD brain wiring. Perhaps you feel as if you're caught in a web that binds you to a limiting sense of yourself in the world. You might wonder if things can be different. The answer is *yes*, absolutely! You can, indeed, live powerfully and proud as a woman with ADHD. You can recognize and begin to untangle the tightly woven tapestry of shame and hiding that contorts your precious sense of self, so that you can step more fully into the authentic and empowered path most meant for you.

Surviving Bravely: Life Before Untangling

When ADHD is undiagnosed, untreated, unmanaged, or misunderstood, the challenges associated with this brain difference are overwhelming. Many of us feel as if we are treading water or barely getting by.

During early stages of living with undiagnosed ADHD, it's likely you felt overwhelmed simply trying to get through the day as unchecked symptoms flared up, "ADHD mind" prevailed, emotional storms overpowered, and every day felt like constant firefighting. There is little room for pride and empowerment when you feel chronically exhausted—both physically and emotionally.

Often at this stage, ADHD differences and the behaviors that result are assumed to be character flaws. Instead of perceiving symptoms as just that, ADHD-related challenges could easily be misinterpreted as some version of the common shame-based story: "I am bad." You might have experienced automatic, critical, even downright mean self-talk as well as intense and uncomfortable emotional experiences during this stage of the journey.

When we try to explain our challenges to other people, it's common to encounter defeating and disempowering experiences of judgment, dismissal, and invalidation. These sorts of interactions fuel negative self-talk, creating a disheartening cycle and more deeply ingrained limiting beliefs. When this happens, our negative thoughts turn into a view of the world that is colored by our internal experiences and beliefs—even if that lens is distorted and those beliefs are hindering.

Because we tend to seek confirmation of what we already believe, the layers add up over time. Living with anticipation of future rejection and judgment can lead to self-fulfilling prophecies and unhelpful, avoidant coping mechanisms. Have you ever stopped seeing friends, lost a week to video streaming, pillaged the cupboards on a search-and-rescue mission, or gone from one glass of wine to a bottle? These coping behaviors serve a function (protection), but they drain your resources and get in the way of engaging in more helpful, ADHD-friendly patterns of thought and behavior.

Discovery: **Are You Surviving Bravely?**

Let's explore the stage of surviving a bit more to see where you are right now. Consider some of these common descriptions of how women feel at this point in their journey and how they might relate to you. Feel free to expand on these.

☐ Swirling, spinning

☐ Dizzy, disoriented

☐ Living in chaos

☐ Chronically stressed, exhausted

☐ Overwhelmed

☐ Going crazy

☐ Barely hanging on

☐ Tangled up, stuck

☐ Lost

☐ On a never-ending roller coaster

☐ Treading water, drowning

☐ Unable to keep up despite best efforts

☐ Alone, misunderstood

☐ _____

☐ _____

☐ _____

Becoming Aware of Your Beliefs

If you don't understand or haven't yet identified your challenges with ADHD, you might be barely surviving day to day. It's understandable that negative self-appraisals and apprehension would follow. Pair this with messages you might receive personally or hear about others—"You're always late," "She only cares about herself"—and you have a recipe for a downward spiral. You might not feel very courageous at this point, but it actually takes a great deal of bravery to wake up and go about the stuff of daily life with persistence and resilience in the face of these hardships. Even in the surviving phase, bravery is present.

What Is Your Self-Talk Really Saying?

Language is a defining part of the human experience and a tool that the brain uses to make sense of things. The way we talk to and about ourselves has profound consequences for how we relate to others, the world, and ourselves. Because adults with ADHD have more negative self-talk than those without the condition, it's important to take a look at how you're talking to yourself (Mitchell et al. 2013).

You might be harboring some version of a common set of fears, beliefs, and old ingrained stories that commonly get translated into self-talk. You might not be fully aware of these thoughts if they cross your mind frequently and automatically. While these thoughts can be rerouted over time and with practice, they must first be recognized without judgment. (Sometimes we even judge ourselves for judging ourselves about judging ourselves! Sound familiar?)

Discovery: Self-Talk Inventory

Below is a list of very generalized and exaggerated negative self-statements that are common among women with ADHD. In particular, these self-statements relate to how you may see yourself, not just your experience of living with invisible differences.

Place a checkmark next to the thoughts you relate to or identify with. After you have read them all, go back and star the three most common for you. Try to do this exercise with openness, compassion, and nonjudgment! And remember, these statements are part of your negative self-talk—and definitely not the truth about you.

- ☐ Something is wrong with me.
- ☐ I am broken and need to be fixed.
- ☐ I don't know if I'll ever be able to have the life I want.
- ☐ I'll never reach my potential.
- ☐ I am unacceptable as I am.
- ☐ I'm a mess.
- ☐ I can't let people know the real me.
- ☐ I must be crazy.
- ☐ I can't do simple things that I should be able to do.
- ☐ I am a disappointment, a failure.
- ☐ I am a lazy slob.
- ☐ I am a burden.
- ☐ I am irresponsible.
- ☐ I am horrible at being an adult.
- ☐ I'm alone.
- ☐ I'm an imposter, a fraud.
- ☐ I'm undesirable.
- ☐ I am too much for other people.
- ☐ I am not good enough.

Reflection: **Exploring Your Self-Talk**

It is possible that, after reading these examples and cues, some more examples unique to your experience have come to mind? If so, expand upon and explore them further here.

_____

_____

When do you notice these thoughts turn up?

_____

_____

Which situations are most triggering?

_____

_____

When you think these thoughts and they feel true, what do you notice in your body?

_____

_____

Which three ADHD challenges tend to be the biggest triggers for negative self-talk?

_____

_____

Describe or draw a situation that makes you feel humiliated, afraid, or as if you want to hide whenever you think about it.

What about this situation was particularly painful?

_____

_____

_____

_____

Understanding Your Identity Triad

ADHD inevitably impacts your sense of identity in these three areas:

- Your core sense of self

- Your feelings about your brain

- Your relationship with the world

When we grow up without an understanding of ADHD or an appreciation for our strengths and differences, our sense of self, our relationship with our unique brain, and our relationship with others get tangled up over the years. The more these three areas become tangled, the more shame multiplies to become a long, weighted knot of secrecy and self-limitation.

Conversely, the more we untangle these three aspects of our identity (core self, brain, and world), the easier it is to begin to decrease the power of our shame and replace it with confidence and a stronger, fuller sense of self.

Because it is difficult to break free of entanglements you can't see or explain, we will start by simply shining a light on the interplay among your sense of self, your feelings about your brain differences, and your relationships with others.

Your Core Sense of Self

Your core *sense of self*, as we mean it here, refers to the unique, nuanced composite of all of the things you are: all of your qualities, quirks, and experiences. ADHD is certainly one part of your core self, and so are your interests, beliefs, values, strengths, challenges, life experiences, and social roles. This is you as a whole person, the big-picture you.

Your core sense of who you are is at the center of everything. It is the essence of your authentic self, the truth of who you are as a complex human being doing the best you can. Your mission, should you choose to accept it, is to form a compassionate, engaging, radically accepting, uncon- ditionally loving relationship with your core self. (Or, let's be real, to have this relationship with yourself more days than not. But hey, shoot for the moon!)

You and Your Brain

The second intertwined layer of your identity as a woman with ADHD is the actual ADHD part: your unique brain wiring. This is manifested in your relationship with your brain, or the ways in which you perceive and support your unique strengths, challenges, and needs. This is where skills and strategies are immensely helpful when applied without shame, judgment, or unrealistic expectations. This journey will help you shed the layers of shame and judgment so that you can honestly, quickly, and compassionately identify, appraise, and engage in supporting actions for your needs as a woman with executive functioning challenges. This one is fairly simple once untangled from the emotional legacy of living with ADHD.

You and the World

Living with ADHD can be tough, and within its inherent difficulties are the seeds for either self-realization or self-constriction. Constriction can occur when our lived experiences as women with invisible differences are infiltrated by shame, fear, and the secrecy generated by stigma. This is further compounded by the presence of additional visible or invisible differences and cultural pressures to conform to unrealistic gender role expectations.

In order to dive into the depths of the internalized messages you have collected over the years about being a woman who has invisible differences, you have to take a leap of faith and believe that living an authentic life of personal power and pride is more important than the fear and pain that have been holding you back.

How Tangles Develop

In order to illustrate how the identity triad can become tangled up, let's take one common difficulty faced by many women with ADHD: disorganization. We can trace this ADHD challenge through the process of becoming tangled up with a woman's core identity.

Tangle #1: The Loop of Shame

Disorganization may be a fact of life for you. However, it needn't be the whole picture. Oftentimes, the problems lay in the tangles themselves. If you struggle with chronic disorganization, you might—at least in certain situations—automatically translate your challenges into self-criticism or shame.

Many women with ADHD are so used to this loop of self-criticism and shame that they rarely notice it happening and are surprised by the frequency and automaticity of their judgment and negative self-talk.

So let's say your ADHD brain causes you to be disorganized. Do you automatically translate a simple description of your brain-based challenge (in this case disorganization) into something broadly self-critical about you as a person? Or maybe you shame yourself, which involves converting something external into an internal, painful core belief about who you are.

In this case, *I have a messy desk/kitchen/car* (you name it!) becomes *I AM A MESS!* This easily turns into *I AM BAD!*

You may be very aware of these automatic thoughts. What you may not be aware of, however, is how these instant self-statements can ensnare and diminish your deeper sense of self-worth and ability to take effective action with compassion and intention in the present moment. In fact, this cycle moves you farther away from being able to manage the symptoms of ADHD (Ramsay 2017). You might become overwhelmed, shut down, avoidant, or even perfectionistic—a recipe for burnout. The inner self-critic may lead you back, time and again, to the "try harder to do it like neurotypicals" mind-set, instead of considering with compassion and freedom what truly and uniquely works for you, what you can accept or release, and where you want support. Over time, these tangles amass and threaten your sense of self.

Tangle #2: The Loop of Isolation and Hiding

Your relationship with others and the world will inevitably be impacted by thoughts such as, *I'm not good enough.* These sorts of internal messages can influence how you let others treat you, how you speak to others and allow them to speak to you, and how you engage with the world in general. Some women begin to isolate and completely hide away due to the shame of being messy (or having another ADHD-related challenge) that permeates to a general belief such as, *I am not worth much to others. I am less than.* Such beliefs illustrate how powerful our thoughts are and how quickly they can affect how we interact with the world and ourselves. At this point, then, *I am messy* has tangled up with your ideas about relationships and taken on yet another unhelpful meaning:

I have a messy desk/kitchen/car, therefore I am bad and should withdraw from others.

Some other common versions of this tangled belief that you might experience are listed below. Keep in mind that sometimes these beliefs operate underneath your conscious awareness. And they can become so ingrained that you don't bother to question them.

I have a messy desk/kitchen/car, therefore:

> *I don't have much to contribute.*
>
> *They can treat me with disrespect.*
>
> *I'm too much for other people and won't be accepted, so why try?*
>
> *I can't be myself around others.*
>
> *I am not deserving of close, supportive, loving relationships.*

If your beliefs about ADHD and yourself are negative, you will perceive the world as a more negative, rejecting, hostile place (Rucklidge et al. 2000). When this happens, you are likely to expect negative outcomes and hide away to protect yourself from the very vulnerability that can actually draw people together.

Reflection: **Describing Your Brain**

We describe our body all the time but rarely think about how we might describe our brain and our experience living within it.

How would you finish this sentence? Consider words such as slow, fast, complicated, broken, interesting, unique, frustrating, spacy, complex, fascinating, and so on.

My brain is: _____

Did you answer through the lens of fear and doubt or from a place of clarity and compassion? Nonjudgmentally notice which words immediately came to mind. Consider adding a few more adjectives to account for the dynamic, complex, nuanced person that you are!

🪷 *Jean's Story:* Trapped and Tangled

Jean felt that she was in crisis: trapped and depressed. She had poured everything into being a wife and mother for three decades. Now that her children were launched and her husband retired, Jean felt that it was time to put herself first, for once.

Jean was diagnosed with ADHD at fifty. Up until then, she had always assumed that she was stupid and invisible because of her undiagnosed brain-based challenges. She put her dreams on hold because pursuing her passions seemed overwhelming amid the responsibilities of managing daily life. With supported exploration, Jean was able to identify the damaging messages she had internalized over the years and the self-talk that played on repeat in her mind every day. I'm such an idiot, I can't do anything right, *she'd hear. The story of being stupid was deeply familiar; it had been there since childhood, when she struggled in school.* I'm kidding myself if I think I can take Spanish classes, *her inner critic would say.* I can't even remember to pick up the dry cleaning! *Jean noticed that her inner critic didn't miss a beat.*

But in the more peaceful moments, Jean knew she wasn't an idiot, even though she had a unique set of challenges. As Jean became aware of her self-talk and its origins, her inner critic became a less credible source of feedback. Instead, Jean was able to consider a kinder, more nuanced view of herself. This, in turn, helped her feel more confident about signing up for that Spanish class. As Jean moved farther from her negative story about her challenges, she was able to move closer to people and activities that enhanced her life.

Reflection: Jean's Story

Which of Jean's thoughts, feelings, or experiences did you identify with?

_____

_____

_____

_____

_____

_____

ADHD-Friendly Chapter Takeaways

❧ ADHD is a genetic, brain-based syndrome that leads to difficulty with executive functioning skills.

❧ Your sense of identity can be negatively affected when your ADHD challenges become tangled up with your sense of self and beliefs about your character.

❧ Critical self-talk and limiting beliefs about yourself further impact your relationships with others and how you perceive and navigate the world.

❧ The untangling process helps you rewrite the narrative of who you are as a whole, worthy, exceptional woman with ADHD.

CHAPTER 3

Dare to Discover

Uncovering Where Damaging Messages About Differences Come From

Women with ADHD grow up knowing, viscerally, that they are different. This is compounded for women of color, those who have a physical disability or difference, those who identify as LGBTQ, those of lower socioeconomic status, or those who otherwise experience daily obstacles and oppression for any number of differences—visible or invisible.

As girls, we learned which behaviors and thinking, learning, and working styles are preferred, which are accepted and tolerated, and which are frowned upon. These preferences were communicated in innumerable ways, from communication streams to public policies and from institutions to our first-grade classroom conversations.

During the course of our lifetime, we as women with ADHD learn through various channels that the way we think, work, speak, relate, and act does not match up with the preferred way of being in the world. In short, we learn that difference is bad. And, because we know that we are different, many of us also come to believe we are bad. As author and psychologist Carol Gilligan (1993, xviii) wrote about the early lessons girls receive, "Difference becomes deviance and deviance becomes sin in a society preoccupied with normality."

Dissecting the unhelpful, dismissive, shaming messages that women with ADHD commonly internalize is complex. The messages we receive about our differences are nuanced and influenced by myriad factors. Language, cultural messages, and life experiences shape us in ways that stretch to the core of who we are—sometimes for better and sometimes for worse. This is why it is so important to do the personal work of identifying, evaluating, and reconstructing our own set of beliefs and biases.

Without going through a process of self-discovery, we risk muddying the waters when faced with the opportunity to correct negative or misinformed messages for ourselves and others. Gloria Steinem (1970) may have put it best in a speech when she said, "The first problem for all of us is not to learn, but unlearn." This is the challenge we embrace when embarking on the journey of untangling.

Invisible Differences and Internalized Messages

There are four major ways you might have acquired destructive messages about your differences that you have internalized:

- You Messages

- She Messages

- Duh! Messages

- Absorbed Messages

These lessons "learned" affect you greatly until you are able to replace them with new, positive, more accurate reflections of who you truly are, even though your difficulties and differences remain.

You Messages

You Messages (as applied to women with ADHD in Solden 2005, 73–74) are direct attacks about your challenges as a girl or a woman that are delivered to you by one or more sources. You might have received negative You Messages about your ADHD differences from family members, friends, teachers, and peers. Perhaps you've been told things like, "You're just being lazy," "You're too sensitive," "You're not trying hard enough," "You're such a mess," or "You could be successful if you'd just apply yourself." These sorts of messages are the easiest to identify and can feel like hurtful jabs to the gut.

You Messages are the result of misunderstanding, misinterpreting, or conflating your character with the behavior that results from your unique brain wiring. Important people in your life commonly have no idea that there is an alternate explanation for the baffling behavior. Their view is so longstanding and ingrained that, by the time you are offered (if ever) another lens through which to view yourself (i.e., an accurate diagnosis!), you might be resistant to shifting your self-view. At that point, you may even think of the diagnosis or explanation as "just an excuse."

Here are some common client examples. Perhaps you can relate to a few:

Sandra's dad always asks her, "Why do you always have to look so slovenly when we are going somewhere important? It only takes a few minutes to get ready and look nice."

A teacher of a teenager commented, "The world won't accommodate you every time you find something difficult."

A professor of a university student dismissed a request for academic accommodations that had been approved by the disability office, nonchalantly remarking, "You're smart! You don't need accommodations, you just need to be more disciplined."

Heather routinely forgets to shut the kitchen cabinet doors and silverware drawers, and to put away the milk. She is unaware of this. Her husband, viewing her through a lens of someone without executive functioning challenges, tells her that he can reach no other conclusion but that she is "inconsiderate, immature, or spoiled."

Discovery: You Messages

Reflect on the effects these kinds of direct messages may have had on your sense of self, your relationship to your ADHD differences, and your relationship to others.

You have likely received many You Messages over the years. Can you identify with any of these?

☐ "You're selfish and don't seem to care about our family."

☐ "You have so much potential, what happened?"

☐ "You have so much to offer if you can just _____."

☐ "You're being lazy and irresponsible."

☐ "It's like you don't even try to do things differently or meet me halfway. It's always the same old thing—and you expect people to keep being sympathetic."

☐ "Your friends aren't going to want to hang out with you if you're always so messy."

☐ "What do you think happens if you're late for a job interview or a date? People will think you're irresponsible."

☐ "What's the matter with you?!"

Which You Messages have been the most persistent or difficult for you?

_____

_____

_____

How do those messages impact you today?

_____

_____

_____

_____

To help you see where some of your own self-talk might stem from, write down memories of any You Messages you received from people in your past. This exercise will help point out the harsh and unhelpful nature of the messages we internalize over the years.

- Family members _____

_____

- Teachers _____

_____

- Friends _____

_____

- Religious community _____

_____

- Colleagues, bosses, officemates _____

_____

- Roommates _____

_____

- Romantic partners _____

  _____

- Peers, schoolmates _____

  _____

- Neighbors, community members _____

  _____

- Others _____

  _____

She Messages

She Messages (Solden 2005, 74–75) are comments that people around you say about women who have difficulties and differences similar to yours, while your secrets stay hidden. This often feels like gossip, as She Messages are not directly addressed to you; rather, they are descriptions of another woman's appearance, behavior, or challenges.

Though these messages are indirect or implied, the latent intimation is received loud and clear: your challenges are unacceptable and dangerous. Even if you are able to "pass for normal" or remain undercover and stay superficially safe, you too experience the cumulative effects of deeply internalized rejection, anxiety, and stress—unable to be truly authentic or receive the support you need to manage your ADHD challenges.

In this way, you learn what is socially preferred and acceptable via indirect communication as much as you might from direct sources. While some messages may not directly comment on your behavior or challenges, they can still hit close to home and leave you wondering, *What do they think about me?…I take meds too—would they date me if they knew?…What if they knew what my kitchen looked like?* In these subtle ways, social groups police the boundaries of acceptable behavior, and you learn that there is a price to pay for the unique way you operate within the world.

We listen to these conversations with trepidation and often say very little or cower away for fear of being found out. These statements might even occur in moments when we are trying to provide support to a friend or loved one who is frustrated with a relationship with someone else. In that moment we are stuck between trying to be supportive and being triggered and afraid. Sometimes we happen to overhear comments from someone nearby, and even though we don't have a deep connection to the person talking, we still feel as hurt as if someone we love commented on our own behavior. Much like when people hear ethnic or misogynistic jokes and don't say anything, we may also not act in accordance with our integrity. We may have an opportunity to speak our truth, but we hold back because we become frozen with hurt and fear. At these times we can feel as if we are betraying ourselves and others.

Here are two short examples of how two different women experienced this.

Kylie's Story: Fear of Being Found Out

Kylie, a young woman trying to fit in with her new in-laws, felt fearful at family gatherings because of the She Messages she encountered there. "Every time someone left the room, there seemed to be comments about how so-and-so had 'let herself go' or was doing something poorly. Since they seemed to judge other women with struggles like mine, I dreaded having my in-laws over. I tried to make everything seem 'perfect' any time they visited. It really wore me down."

Discovery: She Messages

Below are some examples of messages you may have heard about other women who have indirectly communicated a judgment about behavior similar to those with ADHD. Check off ones that resonate and add your own.

☐ "I really thought she had her stuff together!"

☐ "You can bet Nicole is going to forget!"

☐ "It's like she just squanders her potential!"

☐ "Her office is so messy it gives me anxiety!"

☐ "I can't believe Daniella forgot the white-elephant gifts. It's like she doesn't care about anyone but herself."

☐ "Don't bother getting there on time, she's always late."

☐ "Amanda never returns my texts or calls, so why do I bother? Some people are just into themselves."

☐ "I mean, I love Susie, but how is she going to be a dentist?! She's always falling asleep in class!"

🪷 *Donna's Story:* Playing It Safe

Donna worked very hard to keep her desk organized at work, but it took tremendous effort—to the detriment of doing her other important work. Her coworkers didn't know she struggled and, when passing by Donna's workstation, would make fun of another coworker, Wanda, whose work area was covered with a jumble of papers and old soda cans. These comments left Donna feeling like an imposter. She felt as if she were betraying Wanda by staying quiet and not mentioning Wanda's creativity or contribution to the team, and instead safely staying in the closet and changing the subject or slinking out of the room. Donna was learning what women like her can expect to experience if her difficulties were to be observed.

Reflection: What Did You Hear?

What She Messages have you encountered over the years?

_____

_____

_____

_____

Which She Messages have had the biggest impact on your sense of self, your relationship with your ADHD differences, and your relationships with others?

_____

_____

_____

_____

_____

_____

_____

Duh! Messages

The third way women learn negative views of themselves comes as a result of *Duh! Messages,* as in "Gee, why didn't I ever think of that?!" (Note to readers: this is best read in a sarcastic tone!)

These messages come in the form of suggestions such as:

- "Have you thought about making a list?"

- "Have you tried setting a timer?"

- "Do you use a calendar?"

None of these, obviously, are bad or wrong suggestions for a person with ADHD. They are usually just woefully inadequate to the situation facing women with ADHD. When these suggestions are given as "the obvious solution," they not only miss the mark and fail to help but they also communicate a grave underestimation of the difficulty, complexity, and type of problem we are confronting.

These kinds of communications, well intentioned as they may be, can feel dismissive and even belittling. Of course you've thought of these things! You've probably tried these "great ideas" a million times!

This kind of superficial advice, even if well meaning, implies that we are just not trying hard enough or aren't smart enough to see what appears to be an obvious answer to a "simple" problem. Further, these messages covertly communicate distrust that we are able to find solutions on our own. As such, they can be disempowering and inadvertently send the message: "You aren't doing it right." Women want to be heard and believed, without attempts to change or alter our internal experience as we live it.

When you have taken the risk to reveal your struggles in an attempt to connect, seek understanding, or get help, you might have been met with simplified and dismissive messages that convey a need to fix or find a solution to your challenges. This can lead to hiding and demoralization, making it harder and harder to open up and reveal yourself over time. This is because the suggestions you receive communicate a lack of acceptance of your differences, often unintentionally. This might lead you to believe that no one "gets it." You might feel as if you are alone with your challenges, which seem unacceptable to the world around you, and therefore conclude that it is fruitless to bother explaining the complexity of your inner world to other people. (Which leads to, you guessed it: more hiding and withdrawing!)

That's why as you go through this journey, you will see how important it is to move increasingly toward people who see you as a whole, valuable person!

Discovery: "Gee! Why didn't I think of that?"

Below are some common examples of Duh! Messages, to which we have added sarcastic responses for your entertainment—something tells us you'll know what we mean!

☐ "Have you tried using the reminder app on your phone?"

(I only have ten different productivity apps, thankyouverymuch!)

☐ "Why don't you just get in the habit of leaving ten minutes earlier?"

(As if I've never tried to leave early!)

☐ "Have you tried using a planner?"

(Ha! Five this year, actually. Lost three, used one as a color-coding procrastination device, and dropped the last one in a puddle.)

☐ "It's just about staying consistent and sticking to a routine."

(I dream of being able to stay consistent! That's what I'm trying to say is hard for me! Ah! You're not listening!)

☐ "Try setting an alarm to remind you."

(An alarm? To think! That must be what I've been missing all these years!)

☐ "Everyone gets distracted these days!"

(Ugh, here we go! Please just stop talking.)

☐ "Oh, it's not as hard as you think! Try _____."

(Right, but I'm not you! That's the whole thing!)

☐ "Are you getting enough sleep and exercise?"

(Not the exercise thing again! [Eye roll.])

☐ "Maybe you just need to make a few small dietary changes!"

(You know, you're the first to mention this!)

☐ "Just make a list."

(I have a thousand of them on sticky notes all over my house and office. Which one do you think is the magic solution?)

☐ "You're so smart. You just need to think more positively!"

(Never heard that one before. Can you positively think your way out of your chronic health condition, Barb?)

We can all do a collective eye roll now! Any favorites you want to add? Take a stab, it's a good detox exercise. Add as much humor to your private response as possible. Laughter heals, after all.

_____

_____

_____

_____

What are some Duh! Messages that you've received over the years?

_____

_____

_____

How do you tend to respond in those moments?

_____

_____

_____

Is there another way you'd like to handle those comments moving forward?

_____

_____

_____

How have those messages impacted your sense of self, your relationship with your ADHD brain, and your relationships with others?

_____

_____

_____

_____

To the untrained eye, ADHD symptoms can be confusing and misleading, especially if we are seen as highly capable. Others may not understand why we keep "getting stuck" with the seemingly "small stuff" of daily living (i.e., tasks requiring strong executive functioning skills). They assume the answer is practical, simple, straightforward, and behavioral. They often make oversimplified suggestions for strategies that seem like a great "fix" to them.

When the complexity of ADHD is not understood and when these seemingly "simple fixes" don't "work," we can be written off as not trying or following through on their good suggestions or strategies. This further adds to the pathologizing of our differences and challenges, which is difficult to combat. You might not understand yourself what is happening insidiously below the surface. How can you protect yourself internally and interpersonally from this form of assault on your very being while also struggling to understand and accept it within yourself?

The experience of living with ADHD can feel like a lifetime of small assaults, resulting in "the Emotional Distress Syndrome…a chronic state of emotional stress directly related to the struggle to live life with ADHD, a stress that breaks down emotional tolerance, stamina, and the ability to maintain a strong sense of well being and spiritual health" (Ochoa 2016, 44–45).

Absorbed Messages

Mistaken beliefs about ourselves might also have taken root through a more insidious route: by absorbing cultural and media messages or observing the behaviors of neurotypical girls and women to whom we compare ourselves. This may have happened without our conscious awareness, but these constant messages may have colored our ideas about what is expected of women, what is valued in women, and what definitely is *not* valued (like ADHD symptoms).

These sorts of messages about gender roles and cultural expectations are metabolized by us, seeped into our pores from an early age and repeatedly infused into our belief system throughout many years, often outside of direct awareness. This may account for the fact that many women say they didn't receive direct negative messages growing up, so they have a difficult time understanding why they feel shame about their ADHD differences. Messages that are absorbed from the culture and media about what's valued in women are so insidious that the general public often ceases to recognize them—because they are so used to encountering them!

Just like girls and women learn what body type, skin tone, fashion trend, or hairstyle is acceptable through ads, social media, movies, and other modes of cultural indoctrination, we are also continuously taking in concepts of what a woman should be able to do well and naturally. Just like the body shame that we are all familiar with, we also develop shame about the way our brains work. This is something we call *brain shame*.

Due to the unique brain wiring of ADHD, some of the things that women are commonly called upon to do with facility are actually quite complex and challenging for those of us with ADHD. The difficulty occurs in ways that are hard for many to understand, including ourselves!

When internalized gender role expectations meet executive function difficulties, women with ADHD can develop the kind of brain shame that eventually leads to coping mechanisms that keep us stuck, such as hiding, pretending, and avoiding. Explicit gender roles aren't so simple to recognize anymore, since most of us intellectually reject the Brady Bunch mom of the 1970s, yet there are countless scenes, assumptions, and portrayals of what a neurotypical woman does easily and without thought. These conceptualizations of "acceptable" or "desirable" behaviors can be at odds with the sorts of things that women with unique brain wiring struggle with. That's why, early on, we learn how to hide our differences and internalize our shame about them.

> *When internalized gender role expectations meet executive function difficulties, women with ADHD can develop the kind of brain shame that eventually leads to coping mechanisms that keep us stuck, such as hiding, pretending, and avoiding.*

Here is what Olivia, a social worker, says about hiding her ADHD differences and feeling ashamed by her struggles: "I am terribly anxious each time I have to go to the annual Christmas party at a colleague's home. I'm so afraid I'll spill the wine or drop the food, mess up the dish I said I'd bring, bump into someone, or just plain embarrass myself!" Diane, a successful website designer, puts it poignantly: "No one has to tell me that other women do things more easily or better than I do! I have observed this from the beginning of my life!"

Many women with ADHD say that they are truly mystified in one way or another by neurotypical women. They often ask questions such as:

- How do other women do it?

- My sister raises three children, goes to work, makes dinner, goes to the gym, calls her friends, and sends holiday cards on time. I know it's not always easy for her, but it's also not as debilitating as it is for me. I just don't get how she does it. Why can't I be "normal" like her?

- Every time I walk into my friends' and neighbors' houses I'm like, "Where's all the stuff? The clutter and piles and papers?"

We, as women with ADHD, see how other women lead their lives and often feel as if we are, as one woman puts it, "watching a magic show."

🪷 *Sari's Story:* Coloring Outside the Lines

When I was a young girl, I struggled with being able to color inside the lines. I would cover up my picture in art class as the teacher walked around to look and comment. I remember not being able to fold my clothes neatly for inspection at camp. As a young teen, I would try so hard to figure out which kind of knee socks to wear! I wondered why other girls enjoyed going shopping together. As a young woman, I panicked over being asked to participate in the ritual of everyone cooking and cleaning up together on holidays.

Discovery: **Absorbed Messages**

What are some covert sources of idealized messages that you might have absorbed over the years that add to your ADHD shame? Check off ones you relate to. Feel free to expand on these.

☐ Ads, news segments, magazines, or other media sources

☐ Social media feeds

☐ Observing other women function at work, school, or daily life

☐ Hearing stories about how others fairly easily attend to run-of-the-mill tasks, such as getting the oil changed in a car, shopping, participating in regular hobbies, hosting parties, preparing meals, managing finances, and so on

☐ Attending events hosted by neurotypical friends or family

☐ School or work, where you have to fit into traditional modes of learning or working, or be put through great stress to get even small accommodations

☐ The doctor's office

☐ Watching commercials for organizational systems, financial planning, and the like

✿ *Clarissa's Story:* The Road Less Traveled

At thirty-two, Clarissa felt she had hit a wall. As an artist, she was aware that her path would look different from the status quo, but that awareness didn't hold a candle to the fear and feelings of being less than when she was around her peers and family.

Even though Clarissa had begun to learn more about how ADHD impacts her, and even though she had support, she still expressed deep concern that something was terribly wrong with her, that she was inherently flawed. She couldn't manage to keep up with peers who seemed to be surpassing her: saving up for vacations and houses, getting married, finding great jobs with benefits, and so on. She also felt a great deal of guilt that she wasn't able to meet the expectations communicated by her traditional family and community—namely, that she find a job, attend church services promptly and regularly (despite questions about her faith, chronic time management challenges, and a standing commitment to Sunday morning studio time), and search for a husband with whom to start a family. In the midst of the guilt and shame, Clarissa had a hard time determining what she authentically wanted.

Clarissa's large, close-knit family often gathered for large dinners, which were some of the best memories she had as a child. However, she had always struggled when asked to serve in traditionally feminine roles such as cooking, cleaning, and serving. Family members would point out, "Clarissa, this isn't difficult! Your head is in the clouds. Hurry up, people are hungry!" To make matters worse, around every corner seemed to be another relative asking if she had been "seeing anyone" because she isn't "getting any younger" and her parents "are ready for a grandbaby!" Clarissa loved the traditions of her Cuban culture and the laughter and closeness she felt at these gatherings, but as the years passed she felt more and more diminished and lost.

Upon supported reflection with a trusted cousin who understood the nuances of her family and culture, Clarissa was able to explore the various types of messages she had been receiving and internalizing from family, friends, and her community. She began to appreciate the good intentions of her family and feel their caring intent. As discouraging as the actual content of their messages had been, Clarissa's family members were actually trying to encourage her to find happiness in the ways that they, themselves, had internalized as the "right" way. With this in mind, Clarissa was able to acknowledge the messages as separate from her own identity and internal experience, hold gratitude and compassion for the underlying love of her family, and begin exploring what she truly believed and wanted.

Reflection: Clarissa's Story

Which of Clarissa's feelings or experiences did you identify with?

_____

_____

_____

In what way did Clarissa's story remind you of your own experiences? Describe them.

_____

_____

_____

_____

_____

_____

Once diagnosed, Clarissa was able to unlink her character from her quirks, as she realized that there was, indeed, a genetic neurobiological difference that she could not control and did not create that accounted for her challenges. When she took a step back and explored the origins of the messages she had internalized, she was able to begin untangling herself from the web of shame, criticism, and guilt that immobilizes so many women with ADHD.

ADHD-Friendly Chapter Takeaways

❧ You Messages are direct attacks about your ADHD challenges that are delivered to you by one or more sources.

❧ She Messages are not directly addressed to you; rather, they are negative descriptions of another woman's appearance, behavior, or challenges. In this way, we learn what is socially preferred and acceptable via indirect communication.

❧ Duh! Messages are well-intended but invalidating suggestions from others that convey a lack of understanding of the depth and complexity of ADHD and its resultant challenges. They tend to imply that you must be either lazy or stupid to not have thought of such a simple "solution" yourself!

❧ Absorbed Messages are covert suggestions or declarations about the preferred way to be in the world that we metabolize from the general culture, media, and observations of how neurotypical women function. These messages often occur outside of conscious awareness but can lead to deep—and sometimes confusing—feelings of shame about our ADHD differences.

CHAPTER 4

Confront Your Hiding

Acknowledging Unspoken Rules for Women That Made You Hide

Women with ADHD commonly and reflexively engage in self-protective coping mechanisms, the most ubiquitous of which is hiding. In order to move into a brave, bright, bold, and empowered life as women with ADHD, it is essential to uncover, confront, and replace the many manifestations of hiding that are keeping us entangled and alone.

The Causes and Cost of Hiding

Our clients say that the most frequently used coping device to deal with their ADHD "management" is…hiding.

Let's repeat that for emphasis. The coping device most frequently reported by the women with whom we work is *not* a better planner, list-making system, or electronic calendar—it's hiding who they are from other people! We want you to really stop and let that sink in. What does it really mean to manage your ADHD by hiding?

Hiding, when used as a protective device, keeps us trapped from letting the world see who we are. When we hide our challenges, we also hide ourselves as individuals and block our chance to show who we really are, something everyone on this planet longs for. Every single one of us wants to be seen and accepted as we are, in this moment. Women with ADHD want so much to overcome our wounds of invisibility, but instead we keep adding to them by retreating to this false sense of protection.

> *Hiding, when used as a protective device, keeps us trapped from letting the world see who we are. When we hide our challenges, we also hide ourselves as individuals and block our chance to show who we really are, something everyone on this planet longs for.*

You may have started to hide because you didn't feel understood by those around you—or even by yourself. Probably, it was clear to you that your brand of differences was not valued. You may have felt that others couldn't see past your differences, and therefore you were blocked from all that you are and have to contribute. Your intentions have likely been misinterpreted in negative ways. You may have hidden because you didn't want to be "found out"—you heard negative comments about other women with traits or difficulties similar to yours, and you were worried about the price you might pay if the "real" you were discovered.

To begin the process of confronting hiding, it helps to start by looking at your brain-based ADHD symptoms and, subsequently, looking at the process of how they get tangled up and associated with feared consequences, such as rejection, dismissal, or abandonment. This exercise will help you understand how these beliefs may have led you to hide, the choices you made as a result, and the price you have paid.

Discovery: **Brain-Based Symptoms**

Below are common ADHD brain-based symptoms that can lead to the urge to retreat, protect, and hide. It bears repeating that these symptoms are the result of unique brain wiring that can easily become tangled up with mistaken attributions and related fears that lead to self-protecting but counterproductive behaviors—like hiding!

Check off the real ADHD symptoms that you identify with:

☐ Forgetfulness

☐ Disorganization

☐ Inability to accurately predict how long it takes to get things done

☐ Inability to keep track of what needs to be done

☐ Repeatedly needing explanation or restatement of details or instructions

☐ Difficulty speaking in an organized way to express all thoughts

☐ Trouble cooking and shopping

☐ Difficulty with staying on top of daily tasks and keeping belongings organized for yourself, your house, or your children

☐ Messy car

☐ Difficulty keeping up with small talk

☐ Trouble staying attentive during phone calls

☐ Fatigue from a "normal" schedule

☐ Easily overstimulated in stores, malls, or other crowded spaces

☐ Easily overloaded from too much conversation or stimuli, requiring time or space to recover

☐ Trouble sitting still and waiting, even for small or reasonable amounts of time

☐ Blurting out or interrupting during conversations

☐ Other: _____

What is it about your ADHD symptoms that you are most afraid people would think if they "found out" about your difficulties? Check the fears that resonate with you:

☐ I am a slob.

☐ I am lazy.

☐ I must not care enough.

☐ I am self-absorbed.

☐ I am not a good mother, partner, friend, family member, coworker.

☐ I'm not smart.

☐ I'm lost in the clouds, I'm ditzy, I'm a space cadet.

☐ I'm not interested or interesting.

☐ I lack awareness, I'm not sharp.

☐ I'm boring.

☐ I'm not ambitious or motivated.

☐ I'm not dependable, I'm unreliable.

☐ I'm irresponsible.

☐ I'm a complainer, I'm spoiled, I'm entitled.

☐ I am too much for people.

☐ I am too sensitive.

☐ I'm not competent.

☐ I'm worthless.

☐ I'm an imposter, a fraud.

☐ Other: _____

The perceived consequences of being "found out" are powerful triggers to hiding behavior. Check any below that resonate with you.

I secretly worry that I would be:

☐ Laughed at

☐ Left out

☐ Talked about

☐ Yelled at

☐ Disregarded

☐ Devalued

☐ Passed over

☐ Not taken seriously

☐ Not given credit for strengths or contributions

☐ Powerless in relationships

☐ Not listened to

☐ The butt of jokes

☐ Taken advantage of

☐ Abandoned

☐ Rejected

☐ Ostracized

☐ Other: _____

Forms of Hiding

Hiding can take many forms. Sometimes it means staying in the closet for fear of revealing your weakness in a certain area or in front of certain people. Hiding can also take the form of making the choice not to do something you want to, even something that would allow you to use your strengths or pursue your interests!

Reflection: When and How Did You Begin to Hide?

Can you remember a time when it became too risky to make a mistake? Or to take a chance to say what you thought? Or to share that you felt differently? What happened?

_____

_____

_____

_____

_____

What have been the most consistent ways you have chosen to hide?

_____

_____

_____

_____

Can you describe your earliest memories of hiding?

_____

_____

_____

_____

🪷 *Sari's Story:* Whispered Answers

I learned to whisper my answers, rather than speak them aloud, to the person sitting next to me in class, because the risk of being misunderstood or wrong in front of others became too great a risk to take. While this felt more comfortable and safer than speaking up, the drawback was that my teachers never knew that I knew the answers! I had intended to protect myself from possible humiliation should I answer incorrectly or struggle to express myself smoothly, but the result was that I was deprived of getting much-deserved recognition and feedback for what I knew and had to contribute to the class.

🪷 *Michelle's Story:* Sorry, My Place Is Too Messy

Some time in early adulthood, I stopped having friends over to my house for fear of judgment about "the mess." I didn't want to allow people to get too close to my secret challenges. While this protected me from the discomfort of wondering if my friends secretly held judgments or dealing with their criticism, it led to isolation—and my friends began to question my investment in their relationships.

It wasn't until one friend bravely brought this pattern to my attention that I saw what was happening. I hadn't realized that my choice to keep my home off-limits due to organizational concerns was both a protection mechanism and a symbol that unintentionally communicated to others: "Keep out!" This was the exact opposite of what I wanted to communicate, which prompted further reflection and scary but ultimately fulfilling changes.

Discovery: **Holding Back**

Which of these patterns of holding back resonate with you?

☐ I often hold back my thoughts, opinions, and ideas.

☐ I feel like I need to apologize for everything.

☐ I have trouble sticking up for myself and asking for what I need.

☐ I go along with other people's ideas or ways of doing things, even if it means quietly betraying my needs or myself.

☐ I tend to wear a mask and pretend I don't have ADHD challenges so that others don't judge me or treat me differently.

☐ I am afraid for people to know the real me.

☐ I don't take risks at work.

☐ I don't take risks in my personal life, such as attending a new group or class, following up with a new friend, or trying new hobbies.

☐ I don't let people in; I keep relationships superficial or let them fizzle out if they start feeling too close.

☐ I keep people out of my spaces (home, office, car, etc.).

☐ I push away opportunities that might put me in the spotlight.

☐ I don't share my hobbies, talents, or passion projects with others.

☐ I turn down invitations.

☐ I don't ask for help or support.

☐ Other: _____

Reflection: Still in Hiding?

How do you feel during these kinds of hiding experiences (safe, resigned, helpless, sad, frustrated, angry, guilty, neutral, etc.)?

_____

_____

_____

What are you still responding to that makes you hide?

_____

_____

_____

_____

_____

_____

❁ *Irene's Story:* The Annual Girls' Trip

Every year, Irene's sisters and female cousins plan a girls' weekend in a remote location. While the getaway usually sounds nice in theory, on every trip Irene would end up feeling inadequate and trapped. Each time, she would be afraid to decline the invitation because it was a cherished family tradition.

Irene refused to discuss any of her misgivings with the other women both before and during the trip. As a result, not only did she spend the weeks before the annual event filled with dread, but she also spent the entire trip full of anxiety. Irene felt that she didn't have the same skills as the other women for the 24/7 preparations of food, accommodations, planning, and cleaning.

She would became panic-stricken that her "weird" weaknesses would be revealed. For instance, when Irene requested an adjustment in sleeping arrangements due to her chronic sensitivity to noise, she was met with eye rolls from the others for appearing high maintenance and not being able to just go with the flow. Irene would spend most of the weekend in a great deal of internal distress. She refused to discuss her feelings and challenges with even one of the women because she felt so ashamed and fearful of being discovered.

If you find yourself avoiding particular situations, you aren't alone. Below you will find some common examples. What might you be missing out on?

Discovery: Self-Protection

Check off the situations that complete the following sentence:

I don't like or I altogether avoid…

☐ Traveling with others

☐ Driving with others

☐ Working with others

☐ Socializing

☐ Attending gatherings where my difficulties could be revealed

☐ Hosting or cohosting events, even if I secretly would like to

☐ Taking day trips with others to places I'd actually really like to visit

☐ Engaging in hobbies with others

☐ Other: _____

Reflection: **The Price of Hiding**

Hiding exacts a price. Let's discover the toll it may have taken in your life.

What situations would you have liked to share with others but avoided because you were afraid of being discovered?

_____

_____

_____

Describe any opportunities or positions you would have liked or been good at but feared taking the leap to pursue, because they required executive functioning skills.

_____

_____

_____

What have you missed out on because you chose to retreat and hide?

_____

_____

_____

🪷 *Sharon's Story:* Hiding Her "Limits"

Sharon was asked to become chair of an important committee at work because of her excellent ideas and leadership abilities. She was thrilled about being recognized for her abilities, until she realized the kinds of organizational demands it required. Instead of thinking, I am a great fit for this job, which will require administrative assistance, so I'm going to ask for it, she turned down the position. Sharon felt that asking for help would be revealing a weakness that would make others see her for the "limited" person she is.

❁ *Lydia's Story:* Hiding Her Need for Help

Lydia was asked to lecture on a subject she was very interested in and an expert on. However, it required traveling a fair amount. While she enjoyed traveling and the excitement of visiting other great cities, Lydia was not thrilled about the demands this job would place on figuring out how to shop for all the clothes and accessories she would need, packing and unpacking, and keeping up with the myriad logistical and organizational aspects that other women seem to do with ease. She turned down the offer instead of considering creative ways to get assistance with the tasks that she felt would reveal too much "incompetence." Other women don't need this help! *Lydia thought to herself.* I would feel stupid if someone knew I couldn't do this kind of stuff!

Women hide not from judgment itself but from the *anticipation* of pain, disappointment, and disconnection. While it seems that acts of hiding protect us from such discomfort and pain, these protective behaviors exact a large price as we diminish our own light. Instead of blocking and protecting, hiding actually keeps us farther away from what we long for.

Why Women Hide: Gender Meets ADHD

As we have discussed in earlier chapters, gendered mores and expectations are deeply embedded in our psyches. And these norms can and do covertly sabotage women with ADHD by sending us straight into hiding. You see, women with ADHD are not nonconformists out of choice; rather, we have little choice but to deviate from typical roles and social norms due to our brain-based differences. Some of us long to display more traditional gendered behaviors, while others long to break the mold. Women with ADHD, however, don't have as much freedom in making the choice to depart, to stand out, to be visibly divergent from the norm. This conflict can be subtle, but it is deep, pervasive, and not made out of an intentional lifestyle choice.

Roles and Rules

While *gender roles* are agreements about *where* we fall within a group and what responsibilities we hold in it, *gender rules* are guidelines that govern *how* we fulfill our role. These may vary substantially among cultures and in families.

We absorb explicit and implicit rules governing gender roles and conduct while growing up. These "rules" are often internalized with such force that "breaking" them feels punishable by scolding, shaming, or being tossed out of the group. In fact, when one person in a family or group changes or speaks out, it is common for them to receive what are called *change-back messages*, verbal and nonverbal communications to go back to the way things were, where everyone was comfortable, even if the old dynamics weren't healthy or comfortable at all (Lerner 1989, 193).

In healthy families, expectations of behavior of any kind are designed to supply needed structure and security. But the roles and rules are flexible enough to meet individual member's differences and to change as needed to support the growth of each member. While many families more fluidly adjust to these changes, others become stuck in rigid patterns that can be passed down from generation to generation. As a result, the more rigid families tend to develop unspoken and inflexible rules that govern the narrow way the family members operate. The more we understand these rules and their power, the more ability we will have to break cycles of shame and intolerance.

Discovery: Stereotypical Gender Roles in Families

There are several common traditional gender roles that girls, beginning in infancy, are taught and molded to fit and even embrace. (*Yes, believe it or not, this is still a thing!*)

Do any of the following examples sound like roles you played or were encouraged directly or indirectly to follow within your family? Check any that are familiar:

☐ Helpless little girl

☐ Quiet good girl

☐ Caregiver or supporter for parents or siblings

☐ Not very smart girl

☐ Shy girl

☐ Socially awkward wallflower

☐ Other: _____

Intersections of Gender and ADHD

Although gender roles and expectations are not as directly communicated and policed as was the case several decades ago, many women with ADHD feel constrained and restricted by internalized messages about what it means to be a "good-enough" woman in our families, communities, and society as a whole. These implied roles and prohibitions can make it difficult for us to get our needs met—for accommodations, adjustments, or simple understanding and support—and to overcome fears about stepping outside of such constructs. In order to live a bold, satisfying life, it is important for us to become aware of how our ADHD experiences intersect with our experiences of gender and related rules, roles, and expectations.

A fairly simple question such as, "How can I support my ADHD right now?" can easily become "What are the consequences of my asking for help?" or "I need to figure this out on my own and be a team player… What if they think I'm incapable? What if they get mad because I need to set a boundary?… I'll be perceived as angry and entitled. I shouldn't make waves." This further complicates our ability to ask for help, reveal vulnerabilities, and assert our needs to make changes in ways that may affect others.

Pushing back on these prohibitions requires the courage to assert yourself from an empowered space that honors differences. It means taking the risk to break some rules.

Learning to Break the Rules

Laurel Thatcher Ulrich (1976) famously said, "Well-behaved women seldom make history." In the process of unlearning oppressive lessons and untangling from damaging narratives, we are presented with the opportunity to break some rules. This starts with pushing back against what we learned a woman "should" be like.

🪷 *Alexis's Story:* Steering Her Own Ship

Alexis, forty-eight years old, is on the brink of some exciting changes. Tired of working in HR, where she wasn't able to express her strengths and passions, she decided to open her own consulting business with the help of a dependable assistant. Alexis had been dreaming of this leap for years and had finally gotten to a place where she felt strong making the transition.

There was only one thing she dreaded: telling her friends and family, from whom she had withheld this dream for years. After several weeks of working toward confronting this fearful turning point, Alexis came to a therapy session looking depleted and defeated—a drastic change from the week prior. Despite her recent strength and clarity around what she needed, Alexis broke into tears, describing overwhelming feelings of fear, shame, and doubt that she experienced the previous week when faced with communicating her big, exciting dream to others. She said that she had found herself stuck in her head, recalling all of the times when others had called her selfish, emotional, careless, and bossy whenever she spoke up or made independent choices that departed from the crowd.

Growing up, Alexis was considered a strong-willed child. She was outspoken and often came up with her own creative ways of going about tasks—a quality that was not always appreciated by her family members and teachers. She felt shamed and stifled by spoken and unspoken rules about how girls "should" behave. Alexis was terrified that this leap would only reinforce these narratives and that she would be perceived as selfish, impulsive, and overly emotional by those she most needed support from—proving everyone right after all these years.

After talking through these tangles and the ways in which they mirrored internalized messages about both gendered behavior and others' misperception of ADHD symptoms, Alexis was able to recenter herself within her own sense of knowing. As the session came to a close, Alexis asserted what she deeply believed to be true: that not only was she making a good choice for herself and capable of asserting her decision to others, but she was also someone who is capable and worthy of steering her own ship.

Women with ADHD don't necessarily choose to act in nontraditional ways—we simply don't have a choice. We often can't fit into traditional gender boxes because the tasks historically assigned to women often require substantial executive functioning skills—the very areas where women with ADHD struggle. To make matters worse, women with ADHD often say that we have no way of explaining or describing this experience to people who do not have ADHD—regardless of gender orientation. Such gender nonconformity and related challenges are likely to be especially and uniquely layered for members of the trans or queer community, for whom discrimination against gender fluidity is a daily threat to well-being.

Reflection: **Impact of Gender Roles**

What did you learn about asking for help and asserting your needs within relationships that expected traditional gender behavior?

_____

_____

_____

_____

_____

_____

Discovery: **Gender Rules**

We all receive messages about particular rules that proscribe and police the behaviors of women. These rules, and their implied consequences, often get in the way of asking for help or otherwise supporting ADHD brain-based needs.

Do any of the following rules feel familiar to you?

☐ Don't make waves.

☐ Be nice.

☐ Be accommodating.

☐ Don't ask for special favors.

☐ Don't ask for special privileges, such as basic support or appropriate accommodations.

☐ Don't act like you think you are special.

☐ Don't stand out.

☐ Other: _____

Deb's Story: Rules, Roles, and Traditions

Growing up, Deb's family was well regarded in their small community. Her mother, a teacher, was a cornerstone of the school district, always active, outgoing, organized, and in great shape. She fit in well with the other moms in the community and regularly hosted social gatherings, complete with decorations and baked goods. Deb remembered playing kitchen and hostess growing up, and now, as an adult, she longed to replicate her mother's gregarious nature and seamlessly synchronized routine. But she always seemed to fall short.

Deb's father was rarely home. And when he was home, Deb had trouble connecting with him, since she was aware of the unspoken rule to "not add to Dad's stress." She never felt that she could share her true thoughts and feelings or life's natural ups and downs with her father. Deb never felt fully worthy of her parents' efforts and deeply feared disappointing them, so she often hid her challenges to make them happy and proud—and not cause trouble.

Deb learned that women are supposed to be nice and not make waves. When she did find the courage to ask for help or share an opinion, she sensed that she made others uncomfortable. Deb felt like a burden for asking for support, since her unique needs and challenges were quickly dismissed. She felt as if she only annoyed people when she dared to speak up or express disagreement.

Now that Deb lived in an affluent community as a wife and mother herself, she was surrounded by women like her mother—women who were organized, active, on time, wore expensive yoga pants, practiced what seemed to be morally superior parenting techniques, and perfectly adhered to packed schedules. (Quite a setup for a woman with ADHD!) Deb felt vulnerable about her differences when comparing her abilities and challenges to those of the women around her. Although she sometimes idealized the performance of the women in her community, Deb also knew, all feelings aside, that she had some serious differences and struggles that others didn't have and couldn't relate to. It was evident that she was "The Odd Mom Out."

When she tried to keep her challenges a secret and "pass for normal" to keep up with the covert roles and rules in her community, Deb found herself constantly overwhelmed and exhausted—not to mention completely inauthentic. When she couldn't "pass" because her brain-based challenges simply wouldn't allow it, Deb isolated herself so that the women she secretly admired wouldn't discover that she couldn't meet the implied standards for women in her community.

Because Deb grew up in a home where women were responsible for—and excelled at—maintaining connection and rituals in the family, Deb felt particularly pressured and depressed around the holidays. She had internalized a set of rules and roles that she found it extremely difficult to adhere to because of her executive functioning challenges, adding an additional layer of emotional strain. Furthermore, she still felt the pressure of the old family rule that it was inappropriate and selfish to speak up because it might "cause trouble."

Deb deeply believed that her role as "The One Responsible for Carrying on Family Traditions" was nonnegotiable and, as a result, she refused to broach the subject of tweaking these rituals, no matter what it cost her. Deb worried that setting boundaries around her needs and asking for help would disappoint her family and ultimately lead to deep disconnection. These internalized roles, rules, and fears about family traditions and feminine ideals led to tension, stress, and resentment, which made matters worse, often resulting in anxiety and bouts of depression. Deb felt trapped by a lifetime of internalized messages, and she didn't know how to negotiate or navigate them.

Reflection: **Deb's Story**

Do you identify with any of the implicit or observed messages about gender roles, gender rules, or rituals that Deb internalized along the way? How do they impact you?

_____

_____

_____

_____

_____

Breaking the Mold

Regardless of your political identification, most women can relate to the statement by Senate Majority Leader Mitch McConnell to Senator Elizabeth Warren in 2017 that quickly went viral. McConnell, in disagreement with Warren's decision to bypass tradition and speak up on the senate floor, made one of the most poignant public statements heard in a while. "She was warned. She was given an explanation. Still she persisted." This example speaks loudly to the pushback messages women encounter when we go against the grain. Notice that it was Warren's rejection of tradition and use of her voice, not the political leanings or content of her speech, that were rebuked. As women with ADHD on this journey of untangling, we are continually called to persist—against old stories and tough odds.

When women with ADHD come up against brain-based challenges within certain relationships, within settings that rely on traditions embedded with gender roles, or when attempting to engage in tasks traditionally assigned to women (sending holiday cards, baking a casserole for an ill neighbor, organizing the home, etc.), we often experience immense difficulty speaking up to assert our difficulties and needs. We may over-apologize, say yes to requests for favors that we can't or don't want to do, or engage in behaviors that attempt to "make up" for not being able to fit in or otherwise act in neurotypical ways.

You may feel bound by unspoken prohibitions and expectations that further assault your sense of autonomy and agency, effectively silencing you at times when you most need to assert yourself.

Implied Consequences of Breaking Expectations

Along with the spoken and unspoken rules, expectations, and messages about what is preferred within a group, we also pick up on what consequences may lie ahead should we fail to subscribe to the rules. These implied threats can be a tone, look, phrase, or behavior that communicates: "You're going too far. Back down. Go back to the way it was. Don't break out of the mold." These consequences usually insinuate that the well-being of the group or relationship will somehow be at risk if we act in a way that does not conform. We fear that we will be ostracized, judged, and isolated if we speak out or break the mold in any way.

We are often just as reluctant to reveal our strengths or accomplishments as we are to let people see our difficulties. The prohibition is about showing differences, whether these are challenges or gifts. A feared consequence can be receiving subtle messages such as: "Do you think you're better than us?"

Reflection: **Persisting**

Do you remember any subtle prohibitions about showing your strengths or gifts, or breaking from the group in a positive way? How might that have impacted you?

_____

_____

_____

_____

_____

🪷 *Tammy's Story:* You're Full of Yourself!

Tammy is very smart, but she had been underachieving due to her ADHD, which had just been diagnosed. With added support and intervention following her diagnosis, Tammy started pursuing her dream of having her own business. She began to work on creating a new business card and website. She wanted to take some time on Sundays to work on her exciting new endeavor.

The problem was that every Sunday her brothers and sisters-in-law would come over. The women would watch their favorite reality show, laugh, and have fun. But Sundays were Tammy's only time to herself, and she had trouble sitting still for a full television show.

Not only did Tammy feel that she couldn't voice her need for time and space, but she also worried that her family members would make fun of her new ambitions and ideas. After all, they often laughed at her out-of-the-box ideas when she was a child.

Instead of communicating effectively and giving herself permission to claim space to pursue her business, Tammy continued spending Sundays feeling worse and worse. Preoccupied with resentment and trying to keep the secret of her exciting new business and her desire to be elsewhere, Tammy couldn't enjoy the time together the way she would have liked—and she didn't get to do what she really wanted to be doing either. She felt she needed to hide these new parts of herself from the crowd. Tammy was afraid of breaking with the family tradition and having to confront old comments, such as "You're so full of yourself!" Memories of old messages presented a barrier to breaking into her new life.

Because women are primed to nurture connection, we are particularly susceptible to perceived threats to the relationships in which we find meaning or nurturing. And yet, as women with ADHD, we are often forced to do things differently since our brain doesn't always show up for us when we need it to. Impossible as it may be for all women, it is even harder for women with ADHD to live up to the gold standard of the "The Superwoman Imago" (Eichenbaum and Orbach 1987). Having ADHD means that we also are likely to have some unique needs for support, and it can be hard to ask for these things because the act of asking may be a red flag that shakes things up. Sometimes the act of asking is scarier and more problematic than whatever it is we are asking for, especially if we live or work within a system that perceives women's assertiveness as threatening or whining.

Discovery: The Price of Revealing

Have you had difficulty revealing your differences in the past? Check off any of these that sound familiar.

☐ Have you held yourself back from asking for assistance or support in ADHD-unfriendly situations? (*They'll think I'm conceited and entitled. Or they'll think that I think, "I'm special," and then they'll reject me!*)

☐ Have you ever stopped yourself from asking for accommodations (such as asking for flex hours), moving to a quieter area of the office, or closing your door at work, even though you know you could be a much more engaged and efficient team member? (*I don't want to seem unfriendly! I promise I'm a nice person! They will give me negative reviews on my performance evaluation and won't want to get to know me if I do these things.*)

☐ Have you ever wanted to ask for more support staff at work or to suggest to your partner that you get a helper at home, but didn't for fear of the response you might get? (*I already know how this is going to go. They're going to say, "Really? There are more important things to spend money on!"*)

☐ Have you ever had a party and asked people to bring potluck dishes (because you love to entertain but cooking isn't up your alley), only to be met with pushback? (*I really don't want to hear them say, "It's not that hard! Put something in the slow cooker. Cooking isn't rocket science."*)

☐ Have you ever been met with an oversimplified, quietly judgmental response when you've described how overwhelmed you feel when attending baby and wedding showers? (*I really dread hearing, "It'll be fun! Just relax! Have you checked the registry? The good gifts are almost gone!" These things are awful!*)

☐ Have you ever worried about a friend's reaction if you were to ask to have a social gathering at a quiet location outside of your home? (*Technically, I know it's my "turn." I can hear it already: "Everyone else has hosted!" Yuck.*)

Reflection: **The Price of Revealing**

How have situations like the examples listed above continued to affect how you hide or give voice to your differences and needs?

_____

_____

_____

_____

_____

_____

ADHD-Friendly Chapter Takeaways

⚘ One of the most pervasive and damaging coping strategies that women with ADHD rely upon for protection is hiding.

⚘ While acts of hiding appear to serve the function of avoiding discomfort, conflict, and vulnerability, they also lock away much of who you are and what you have to offer the world.

⚘ Hiding takes you out of your life.

⚘ Gender roles, rules, and expectations add fuel to the fire for women with ADHD, as they further complicate and impede attempts to assert your voice, take up space, and unapologetically stand by your unique needs, preferences, ideas, and strengths.

⚘ The ultimate effect of self-silencing and reinforcement of hiding behaviors adds yet another barrier to your attempts to create a life that supports your ADHD challenges and highlights your strengths.

PART II

Brighter

"Most of the shadows of this life are caused by standing in our own sunshine."

—Ralph Waldo Emerson

As Emerson eloquently alludes to in this quote, our biggest obstacle to overcome on the path to change is fear of our own light. Emerson's reflection speaks to the periods of hardship and darkness that we contribute to, and perhaps even create, by resisting our own right to shine.

Shining—allowing ourselves to envision and step into a brighter way of living as women with ADHD—requires us to consider what we truly want, to show the world more about who we are, to choose with whom we want to connect, and to admit from whom we may want to move away. This process may trigger internal barriers that run counter to what we learned as girls about how women are expected to behave in accommodating ways.

Women with ADHD commonly express fears and encounter resistance on this leg of the journey. Which is why this entire section, Brighter, is dedicated to helping you walk across the bridge that leads to stepping out of your own shadow and onto the path most right for you.

Now is the time to focus on imagining a whole new vision of yourself and trying out a new version of your life as a woman with ADHD. So let's continue, *brightly*.

CHAPTER 5

Adjust to Brightness

Playing with Possibilities

Marianne Williamson, a famous inspirational author, expressed a similar sentiment to the Emerson quote at the beginning of this section when she wrote, "Our deepest fear is not that we are inadequate. Our deepest fear is that we are powerful beyond measure. It is our light, not our darkness, that most frightens us" (1996, 190).

Williamson's quote is particularly powerful in light of the journey you are taking as a woman with ADHD. Like most people, you might find yourself feeling uncomfortable, ill prepared, and overwhelmed when the clouds part and warmth or opportunity enters your life.

The very idea of the sun shining on you might feel too unfamiliar and bright when you are used to keeping your head down, just trying to survive with the ever-changing weather of your atypical brain and fluctuating emotional space. Growth, change, and stepping more fully into your own light might feel utterly implausible, perhaps even irresponsible. If you are not ready for unexpected brightness, your first impulse might be to turn away or cover your eyes. You might retreat inside.

At this point on your journey, however, it is likely that going back into the darkness of hiding no longer feels as safe and tolerable as it once did. So, hopefully, you will consider adjusting your plans. Instead of retreating, maybe this time you can take a moment to regroup, grab some sunscreen and a floppy hat for protection, and let yourself step outside to bask in the warmth of the sun.

We want you to understand that for most women, ADHD or not, considering the possibility of shining more brightly can trigger fear and doubt. Change brings up anxiety about a lot of things, not just about ourselves and whatever happens to be shifting in our life but also about how other people in our life might react. This is a normal and expected part of the process; it is an inevitable and necessary component of this kind of transition. Remember, it not only you who is changing! As a result of your shifts, everyone else in your orbit will have to adjust, and that will take some time and persistence. We encourage you to be patient with the process.

With ADHD, there have always been missing pieces of the jigsaw puzzle that make up the whole picture of yourself. Now is the time to begin thinking about constructing a new image of yourself that puts back the missing pieces or corrects the image to make it more complete and accurate after years of distortion and discouragement. This more complete and accurate image of yourself and your possibilities has to include an integrated understanding of your strengths and your challenges, as well as your interests, needs for support, resources, and, especially, the enduring character traits you possess that you can depend upon.

When we have the vulnerabilities of ADHD, we are usually acutely aware of our difficulties. Yet our core traits that are natural and enduring are often overlooked because we view them as "no big deal" or "just part of who I am." ADHD symptoms and experiences can easily dominate our view of ourselves. We might take our strengths and core character traits for granted. When we overlook these enduring core traits, we don't have a chance to build on them, and so we can't develop a sense that we can count on the foundational parts of ourselves when we need them most.

Trying On New Dreams

This stage of the journey into brightness is about trying on new ideas, stories, and visions in the same way you might experiment with new styles of clothes: by having fun and knowing that you aren't making any commitments yet. You may laugh and discard most of what you try on, but, since you let yourself be open to possibilities, you might actually find a few new items that reflect who you truly are now.

In the same spirit of fun and playfulness, let yourself enjoy taking out some old dreams to see how they fit. Decide what needs to be altered, discarded, updated, or stored away to forever remain a cherished fantasy. Playfulness is the key to "resisting the resistance" to your expanding narrative and to letting down your guard.

Dressing Up Your Hopes and Dreams

In order to begin to update your old dreams, it is helpful to identify what kind of dreamer you might be and to discover what your relationship to your most cherished, discarded, or undiscovered dream is. Most of us had dreams early on as children. Some were fantasies built on superheroes or our parents, what we saw on TV, or a favorite teacher or aunt. For some of us, early dreams were based on discoveries of real talents or passions. This may have led to years of nurturing secret hopes and dreams about fulfilling them. For others, dreams were put aside early because our circumstances in life were harsh and didn't allow for the kind of privilege or luxury of pursuing them. And still others may have found ourselves drowning in the details of daily life to the point that our dreams and hopes eventually became lost at the bottom of our piles.

For women with ADHD in the early phases of adulthood, there is often a sense of being lost, discouraged, and completely uncertain as to how to proceed toward our (or any) vision of the future. Many are not sure where to begin or have trouble identifying their dreams, passions, and interests in the first place.

Jennifer, a client, wrote to us:

> For me the issue is not just about getting organized. It's about the feeling that I don't have the right to hope and dream.

This statement depicts the pernicious nature of lost hopes and dreams that is common among women with ADHD. And this loss of hopes and dreams can slowly kill off our spirit, drowning out our feelings of vitality and aliveness. A feeling of purpose is an essential ingredient that drives human beings and combats hopelessness. Therefore, discovering a sense of purpose and making meaning from life experiences is a pivotal element of successful treatment of adults with ADHD.

The key measures of effectiveness of treatment have to go beyond whether an individual has increased punctuality or decreased the size of her piles. While strategic support of specific ADHD symptoms and challenges is necessary, comprehensive treatment of ADHD also needs to include questions such as: "Am I moving toward a feeling of greater authenticity and meaning, and am I realizing the hopes and dreams that make me feel alive?"

Compelling visions and a sense of purpose stimulate and activate us, which is crucial for adults with ADHD whose brains crave and require input that is highly stimulating. Exploring what gives us purpose, meaning, and future direction isn't just a bunch of feel-good fluff—discovering what lights us up is imperative to regulating the ADHD brain.

> *Compelling visions and a sense of purpose stimulate and activate us, which is crucial for adults with ADHD whose brains crave and require input that is highly stimulating. Exploring what gives us purpose, meaning, and future direction isn't just a bunch of feel-good fluff—discovering what lights us up is imperative to regulating the ADHD brain.*

Four Types of Dreams

When you look at your early dreams, you may find that you want to take some off a shelf and dust them off, while others you feel are treasures to keep forever in a special memory box. Whatever your relationship is with your earlier dreams, it is important to discover how they fit you now so you can consider what you want to do with them.

Think about what happens when you go through the clothes in your closet (a dreaded ADHD task). You might feel overwhelmed at the thought of weeding through all those old clothes. Some pieces might make you feel discouraged since you don't fit into them anymore, while others might make you feel nostalgic for a beloved time in your past. Other pieces you come across might surprise you because they had been stuck in the back of the closet and you had forgotten all about them. When you look more closely, you see how they can be altered and updated to fit you at this moment in your life. You may also realize that there are many pieces of clothing you are ready to let go of. Even though it may have been a grueling process at the beginning, by the end of this discovery and sorting process you are likely to feel lighter, freer, and more relaxed.

In the same way that you update your wardrobe, you can go through your old dreams and sort them into four mental boxes:

- Save But Needs Alteration

- Needs an Update

- What Was I Thinking?!

- Discard and Start Fresh

SAVE BUT NEEDS ALTERATION

When we examine old childhood, teenage, or early adult fantasies or dreams, we often find some that are completely outdated. Certain elements, however, may still fit in some ways but need to be altered for the current phase of life. In this box go dreams that still fit and speak to your talents and passions, but need to be altered to adapt to who you are now.

🪷 *Margi's Story:* Born to Sing

When Margi was a teenager, she was a pretty good singer and was in a school band. She even had dreams of becoming a Broadway star. Now forty, she has come to terms with the fact that she is past the stage in life when becoming a Broadway star is possible. She hasn't sung in public since high school, even though while she is in the shower or driving she sings out loud with passion and secretly thinks she is still "pretty good."

Since Margi has been diagnosed with ADHD, treated with medication, and joined some online groups where she connected with other women with ADHD, she is beginning to feel more sure of herself and wants to prioritize her time and energy in ways that are more satisfying. Margi realizes that elements of her early dream still speak to her.

Margi worked with her ADHD coach to figure out how to transform her youthful dream of performing into her current stage of life. Instead of just leaving her dreams in the past, gnawing away at her every time she sees someone sing in public, Margi worked on fulfilling her earlier dreams and desires—but in an altered form. She began to take singing lessons. She eventually got the courage to sign up for a talent show at a national ADHD conference, where she sang for a very supportive crowd who cheered her on, even when her voice quivered. She was encouraged by the reinforcement of her peers and felt invigorated walking off the stage.

Eventually, Margi joined a local theatrical group through which she is able to sing in productions of the Broadway shows she loved and dreamed about being part of when she was a teenager.

Reflection: Save But Alter

"My old dreams were true then and are still true now. They are based on strengths or talents I actually had or have and still want to fulfill in my life in some form." Does this statement ring true for you?

☐ Yes

☐ No

Which parts of these early visions still spark you?

_____

_____

What would be a form of these visions that might make sense for you today, at this time in your life?

_____

_____

_____

_____

NEEDS AN UPDATE

Some pieces of our dreams were never based completely in reality but instead represented a core element of our personality that we wanted to express in some way. The meaning of the dream still remains but the actual form doesn't matter as much as what we wanted to express.

In this case, we may need to understand what the meaning of a particular dream was even if the original form wasn't based on true talents or desires (Solden 2002). Maybe you liked the idea of being a rock star even if it was never realistic and you couldn't carry a tune or keep a beat to save your life—yet, there was something inside of you that has always wanted to stand out and be listened to and admired. Maybe what still lives in you—what remains core to you—is a desire and latent ability to express yourself, to be seen, or to be in front of people who will listen to you. Maybe you long to let loose in some way you have not been able to do during all these years of struggle as you tried to control your life with ADHD.

✿ *Jamie's Story:* I Want to Be Seen

Unlike Margi, who actually wanted to sing and had the voice to back it up, Jamie wanted to sing but couldn't carry a tune. As a young girl with ADHD of the predominantly inattentive presentation, she was perpetually lost in thought and was shy. She thought that maybe she wanted to act or sing or dance, but, as a young adult looking back on her childhood, she realized those weren't actually true interests or dreams. What Jamie always really wanted was to be seen and heard. Her true dream was to have confidence and let people see how smart and creative she was—instead of hiding safely in the background.

Jamie was in her midtwenties when she was diagnosed and began working with a therapist. She had been feeling very lost, discouraged, and anxious. Even though she felt better after beginning treatment and understanding her challenges, she was still unsure how to proceed. When she began to examine her early dreams, she realized that the core meaning— being seen and heard—was still very much alive and that she still longed to fulfill that fantasy.

With support, she joined a public speaking group with whom she practiced reading essays aloud. She gained confidence and went on to find her voice at work, where she began making creative presentations in front of groups. She was finally recognized for being the creative young woman she had always been.

Reflection: Needs an Update

"My old dreams were more of a fantasy. They were more representations of qualities or experiences that excited me rather than realistic goals. But the elements of those dreams still resonate, and I want to understand them more so that I can pursue them in some way." Does this statement ring true for you?

☐ Yes

☐ No

What did your old dreams represent? What themes or desires stand out?

_____

_____

_____

Can you think of a way to reenvision the threads of your early dreams into your current life in a way that fulfills the purpose of your original dream?

_____

_____

_____

WHAT WAS I THINKING?!

As if we are going through a pile of old clothes, when looking through our old interests, dreams, and goals, we might ask ourselves, *Wow, what was I thinking when I bought all these? I didn't have a clue! I don't like any of these anymore. They never really expressed who I was!* Many of us with ADHD say we never had a clear image of our future. Even if we had dreams or wishes at one time, those ideas seemed more the stuff of fantasy than reality.

Maybe you never asked yourself questions about what you wanted. Maybe your life path and ADHD symptoms went off track in unanticipated ways that derailed your original intentions. Maybe you could never figure out what you wanted to do, no matter how many times you asked yourself or bounced from one thing to the next without ever feeling that extra-special pull. Perhaps you haven't let yourself have dreams. Maybe you believed that thinking of such things was a luxury that you didn't deserve or have time for in light of other life demands and circumstances.

🪷 *Eliza's Story:* A First-Time Dreamer

Eliza had a tough life. In addition to undiagnosed ADHD, she was raised by her grandmother and always had to work to help out. She was easy to miss as the bright little girl she was because she was always disorganized, always losing her belongings. She struggled to stay awake at school because she never got enough sleep. Determined to get good grades, Eliza would stay up late to study, even though she had to take care of everything around the house, as well as hold down an after-school job as a teenager.

She felt anxious much of the time, but no one knew how much she struggled or how much she overworked. Her focus was on helping her grandmother and herself survive. She wanted to please her teachers and grandmother by getting good grades, but no one helped her envision her future, and no one helped her understand her challenges. Although she started community college after high school, she eventually had to drop out to earn money for the family. In addition, the writing and reading demands became too much for her.

Eliza stopped asking herself the important questions and moved on with life. Twenty years, three children, two husbands, and many boring jobs later, when her child's doctor diagnosed her son as having ADHD, he turned to Eliza and asked, "Have you ever thought that maybe this answers some of the questions about your life as well?"

Eliza was properly diagnosed, went on ADHD medication, began to read about women with ADHD, and, after all those years of feeling depressed, began working with a counselor. Eliza was speechless when the counselor asked her, "Eliza, what do you want?" She had no idea. She had not asked herself these questions for a very long time. She was exhausted from just coping all these years. She had no idea what she had ever wanted or how to begin to answer that question now. "What do I, Eliza, want?"

Reflection: What Was I Thinking?!

"I never had a dream, or I have had many dreams but they were constantly changing and none really took hold." Does this statement ring true for you?

☐ Yes

☐ No

How can you make space in your life to try out new notions and experiences?

_____

_____

_____

_____

_____

What is one thing you'd like to explore but haven't set aside the time or resources to do so?

_____

DISCARD AND START FRESH

Have you ever had the experience of looking at your wardrobe after you have had a big change in your lifestyle or career and decided that they just don't match who you are anymore? Perhaps you wore some of the outfits to important and memorable events. Maybe some bring up a great deal of nostalgia, but you know that you are a different version of yourself now and it's time to let go.

Even though your earlier dreams may have been fulfilled, things may have changed dramatically and you need a whole new approach. This happens when people retire, switch careers, or move to a completely different area. You may look at your wardrobe and think, *This was a great wardrobe ten years ago. I am a different person now.* Or *I used to stay at home with my little children and now I am a corporate lawyer.* Or *I used to be a corporate lawyer and now I'm an artist living in the country.*

In this same way, you may have actually found fulfillment of early dreams at another stage of your life, but now things have changed. This could be through the death of a partner, a major illness, a move to a different part of the county, a remarriage, a change of jobs, loss of a job, a new child, new interests, and so on.

Now that you have been diagnosed and treated and healed some wounds, you might be ready to develop sides of yourself you never even knew you had the ability to focus on because of your ADHD. It may be true that you may have, by now, outgrown old ideas of who you are and what and who you can be in the world.

🪷 *Laura's Story:* New Dreams for a New Life

Even though Laura always dreamed about being a teacher when she was young and fulfilled this dream, many years later she found that she needed a new dream. She got married, moved to England with her husband for a year for his job, and realized there was an entirely different side to her that she was able to finally pay attention to.

Laura needed retraining, since the world of technology had changed so much, and decided to take classes in web design, for which she found she had a natural ability. When she returned home she changed careers and began developing websites for businesses—with the help of an assistant to keep track of customers and orders, of course. Even though she had loved being a teacher, the pressures of working in the school system were always a source of terrible strain for her. Now she was ready to be in a different field and working with adults.

Reflection: Discard and Start Fresh

"So much has changed in my life. I'm far from the person I once was, and I can't relate to my old dreams." Or "I have already achieved my dreams as much as I care to. It's time to start over." Does this sound like you?

☐ Yes

☐ No

What are the more interesting elements of your experiences or contributions up to this point that you'd like to weave into something new?

_____

_____

_____

In the service of pursuing other things, are there parts of dreams that you let go of that you want to return to and develop now? If so, explore and describe them.

_____

_____

_____

Dream Awakener or Dream Catcher

It is critical that you find the space and time to let yourself begin to develop your dream and to let those new visions take shape. Like those old Polaroid pictures that slowly developed before your eyes, you too may have to wait until the image of your dream appears. This will require you to claim some time and space emotionally and mentally to let yourself wander around the world of possibilities.

The first step to getting in touch with yourself and formulating a vision of any type is to find a quiet space where you feel comfortable and safe and are unlikely to be disturbed. You might find that you have to practice this sort of quiet envisioning in small chunks of time to begin with, building as you go, since this work will require you to step away from your usual routine to let your mind explore and imagine in a relaxed way.

This kind of calm, purposeful distractibility (also known as creativity!) might be unfamiliar or uncomfortable to you, especially if you are used to trying to micromanage your ADHD brain. This is an opportunity for you to enjoy spending some time with yourself, allowing your mind to wander. Don't let yourself get caught up in thoughts of *But…, That's not practical…, I can't…, That would never happen…,* or *How would I pay for that?* Invite the distractibility for once; use it to dream!

Finding a Space to Awaken or Catch Your Dreams

Every woman with ADHD has unique needs and preferences when it comes to finding spaces that are soothing and allow the mind to wander with ease. Perhaps there is a café that you like or a new coffee shop you've wanted to try. Maybe there is a nook or room in your house that you can turn into a private retreat with small, nourishing pleasures such as candles, pillows, blankets, and music.

Is there a friend or family member who would be supportive of your taking time alone and who might offer the use of their home, or a room in their home, as a sort of personal retreat? Maybe there is a friend who'd be willing to join you at a bed-and-breakfast, where each of you could have some alone time but come together for meals or a simple activity. If it's nice outside, consider finding a table in a park or laying out a blanket somewhere in nature. Even the bathtub will work if that is the only place you can manage. The key is to find a space that will help awaken your ability to dream.

Finding Time to Awaken or Catch Your Dreams

For some, daydreaming and exploring come very naturally. For those with inattentive traits, however, this sort of intentional daydreaming might seem a bit risky, because it may have gotten you into trouble before. For others, allowing time and openness to take space for yourself and work through a process of envisioning can be difficult or even unappealing, because you are exhausted from ADHD life or simply prefer more "rational" approaches to problem solving.

Whatever your relationship to dreaming, it's important that you try this activity. Start with just a few minutes at a time. Then build up to ten minutes a day or an hour per week. Or you might take an hour or two right away! You say you don't have time? You can do these imagination exercises in the shower!

With ADHD, it is essential to consider your unique fluctuation pattern of mental and physical energy throughout the day, as well as where and when you have the least amount of distractions and interruptions.

Ideas might also be triggered (at any time) from a special book of inspiration, from a new journal or sketchbook, or by recalling internal visions you have had. Simply allow yourself to pause on them a little longer than usual.

Discovery: **What Sparks You?**

Here are some more ideas for collecting and recording your awakened dreams. Do any sound plausible to you?

☐ Use the notes app or voice recording function on your smartphone to record an idea or experience you had that you might want to re-create or build upon.

☐ Take photos of objects and places that intrigue you.

☐ Follow social media accounts of people and organizations that inspire or encourage you.

☐ Make a Pinterest board of ideas, images, and resources related to an idea or possibility.

☐ Keep a journal for writing, drawing, collaging, or otherwise depicting various facets of ideas, dreams, and future visions.

☐ Tear out magazine pages with stories or images that spark your interest and put them in your daily line of sight.

Following the Threads of Connections

Sometimes it isn't until we look back that we can put all the pieces together. Usually there are threads that connect our earliest stories to our lives much later. This is true even for us, your authors. Here's what we saw when we recently looked back at the threads that have always run through our lives that have led us to what we do today and how we understand our stories at this point.

❋ *Michelle's Story:* Connecting Childhood Dreams to a Career

In third grade I was asked what I wanted to be when I grew up. I said that I wanted to be a teacher, a writer, or a pianist—meaning piano player, which is something my classmates mistook for something else, because…kid jokes. I was terribly embarrassed at the time. I felt that I sounded stupid and shouldn't bother to think of such silly things, let alone share them with my peers. I always seemed to be the odd one out; everyone else gave "normal" answers like nurse and firefighter, but I had to say pianist!

Not too long after, ADHD got in the way of following through on becoming a pianist. I struggled to practice consistently and forgot things I had learned thoroughly. So, understandably, the piano and lessons went away and I was quickly on to the next interest.

For many years, I wanted to be a teacher or a writer. After all, teachers liked me and books make for great friends. I thought about becoming a vet, because animals are both cute and unconditionally accepting. And then, in middle school and into my early high school years, my dreaming came crashing to a halt.

My ADHD was undiagnosed at the time, and I was struggling with feelings of inadequacy, shame, and confusion about my unexplained challenges. Who cared about future dreams when I could barely get through the day? I was fortunate to have access to help, hobbies, and people who believed in me when I didn't. I began therapy with a woman named Mary, who helped me see myself as whole and capable. I started dreaming again.

It was because of Mary that, at fifteen, I said I would become a psychologist. After all, I had something to prove to myself, and when a woman with ADHD has a deeply personal cause, watch out, world! Completing graduate school is the biggest, most

> *Sometimes it isn't until we look back that we can put all the pieces together. Usually there are threads that connect our earliest stories to our lives much later.*

meaningful goal I have ever followed through on; it helped me learn that I can trust myself in spite of my challenges.

What both baffles and moves me tremendously is that, when I look back, a lot of the dreams I had as a child and adolescent stayed with me and actually manifested in indirect ways—even when I thought they were long gone or felt unworthy of pursuing them. Part of what I do now involves teaching, reading, and public speaking, so in some ways I did indeed become a teacher. I loved nonprofit work in college, and now I work closely with the Attention Deficit Disorder Association (ADDA). I also became a writer, and, obviously, I became a psychologist.

This is all to say that sometimes we, as women with ADHD, have dreams that we don't even recognize as such, that we don't allow ourselves to fantasize about enough to acknowledge that maybe even just a fraction of those early childhood dreams have come true or still have the chance to do so. I assumed that becoming a psychologist meant I was turning away from being a writer, a teacher, a nonprofit administrator, and a creative. I was scared that I couldn't "handle" my biggest dreams and might not be able to bring forth the various parts of myself and my life that I value most. It wasn't until I purposefully looked back at my childhood dreams that I realized I had actually, unintentionally, walked straight into them. I might have been scared of my dreams and doubted my ability to achieve them, but there they were, all along.

❀ *Sari's Story:* The More Things Change…

One of my earliest memories is as a six-year-old sitting at a table overlooking a rose garden in my room, writing simple stories about becoming a psychiatrist and helping a little girl who was afraid of dogs overcome her fear. When I was little, I used to watch the Academy Awards and dream about that kind of success. I spent my preteen years dancing around the living room to Broadway music and singing and acting out the parts.

What do those mean for me looking back now? I definitely always had a need to express myself, either in front of people or through writing, and I always had a desire to help people with their struggles. I found out by the third grade that I couldn't carry a tune when they asked me to just mouth the words in music class! So I had to channel some desires in a new direction.

Even though I took radio and television classes in college, I eventually turned to mental health and writing and speaking in front of people about my ideas. I had to keep molding my visions to reality, but I also had to keep moving toward an increasing sense of authenticity.

Discovery: **Early Ideas About Your Future**

Here are some roles that are often incorporated into early dreams and visions of the future. Check any that strike an old chord or resonate as still alive.

☐ Rock star

☐ Journalist, author, writer

☐ President, government official

☐ Documentary filmmaker

☐ Soccer star, athlete

☐ Teacher, professor, coach

☐ Nurse, doctor, paramedic

☐ Mentor

☐ Mother

☐ Musician

☐ Actor, performer, comic

☐ Counselor

☐ Caretaker of people, plants, or animals

☐ Designer of fashion, interior spaces, or graphics

☐ Artist, illustrator, painter, jewelry maker, potter

☐ Chef, baker

☐ Librarian, book store clerk or owner

☐ Architect, construction worker, builder of interesting things

☐ Advocate, lawyer

☐ World traveler

☐ Veterinarian, zookeeper, companion to animals

☐ Leader of some sort

☐ Public figure or speaker

☐ Other: _____

Reflection: **Connecting the Dots**

If you are still coming up blank, these prompts may help you remember your original dreams and discover kernels that might still be alive inside you.

Can you find a thread of connection between your childhood dreams and experiences and your life up until this point? What might it be?

_____

_____

_____

What lessons or experiences have your detours given you that you are grateful for, that you probably wouldn't have learned or experienced in other ways?

_____

_____

_____

_____

_____

_____

❀ *Jessica's Story:* Curiosity Saves Her Life!

When Jessica was a child, she was interested in everything. Her parents used to say to her jokingly, "Remember, Jessica, curiosity killed the cat!" Jessica's parents were both doctors and they never hid their aspirations that their only child, a bright little girl, would follow in their footsteps.

And, indeed, Jessica was interested in science—and math, and soccer, and dress designing, and her friends, and running for class president, and reading. She dreamed so many dreams! She would be a famous scientist who would discover a cure for AIDS. She would help earthquake victims in foreign lands. She would be an astronaut, the first woman president. Clearly, Jessica was not lacking in big dreams! She just had a lot of them and wanted them all.

In her teens, Jessica excelled in most of the subjects that were interesting to her, but she was mostly lost in undiagnosed ADHD instead of practical application of the material. When it came down to choosing a college, Jessica had a terrible time. She had no idea what she wanted but eventually chose a liberal arts college, where she would have more time to explore and decide.

As ADHD fate would have it, when it came time to pick a major, Jessica struggled. She didn't know why she had to pick just one thing and changed majors several times. What she really wanted was to put together an interdisciplinary degree that combined all her interests! She came up with an independent study program wherein she could study abroad as a health professional overseas while helping local women start small businesses, such as farming and selling crafts. Her academic advisors were not similarly impressed.

Jessica eventually graduated, a few years behind schedule, with a major in physics and a minor in sociology. She thought about going to graduate school but the pressure was just too much—and there were too many interesting things to pursue. Once again, she was lost in ADHD indecision.

Jessica took a year to work in an urban setting tutoring children in math and science. Then she met Matt, and they were off traveling around the country for his career. Jessica and Matt had two children, and Jessica became the most creative room mother and PTA president in the school's history.

By the time her children were teenagers, Jessica found herself feeling empty and somewhat depressed and resentful. After talking to her psychiatrist about antidepressant medication, she was surprised when he diagnosed her with ADHD and put her on medication for that. It was then that Jessica began working with a therapist and started pulling together all the threads of her life and talents. She went through a full battery of psychological testing, and the assessments showed that while she had difficulties with attention, she was also exceptionally smart! This is often called twice exceptional, *which means a person has some challenges, such as ADHD or a learning disability, while also testing as very smart, or gifted. This perplexing gap between abilities and challenges can cloud the picture and make it so that people who are twice exceptional are unidentified and misunderstood, so they don't always get the help they need.*

This understanding changed Jessica's view of herself and her life. When her children went to college, so did she! She figured it was her turn to fulfill her own dreams and talents. She enrolled in graduate school in public health and eventually became involved in designing a program that helped women in developing countries start their own businesses by selling what they sewed and created.

ADHD-Friendly Chapter Takeaways

🪷 Practice imagining, playing with possibilities, expanding options, and trying on new ideas of *you*, like those old childhood games of dress-up and make-believe.

🪷 Begin to reawaken, capture, alter, or update your early dreams to give you a compelling future to move toward.

CHAPTER 6

Restore Wholeness
Moving Toward an Authentic Vision

We can begin to see ourselves as whole, complex human beings—instead of in pieces or incomplete, or from a distorted point of view. This is not sugarcoating the struggles of ADHD. This is not saying ADHD is a gift in itself. It's not so black or white, good or bad, all or nothing. Rather, this perspective is saying, "I have many parts that make up who I am, as do all human beings. Mine might be a little more difficult to put in a neat little bundle or cohesive self-picture, but now that I am diagnosed and have that piece, I can begin to understand the other parts of me that have been masked, ignored, misunderstood, or just plain missed all these years."

This idea is a lot to take in. The process of seeing ourselves whole unfolds over time. Once we recognize, understand, and accept our natural resistance to change, we can feel calmer about going forward.

Lorraine is a good example of the change that can happen when we begin to see ourselves as "whole."

Lorraine's Story: I Hated Going to Parties

Lorraine, a teacher, despised going to parties because she inevitably bumped into tables, spilled wine, forgot what she was saying midsentence, dropped food, and generally felt embarrassed and hopelessly inadequate. Her ingrained response when this happened was to profusely apologize and put herself down. By putting herself down before anyone else could, Lorraine felt as if she were protecting herself.

But this position was ultimately hurtful, because it didn't do anything to help Lorraine feel strong and project confidence. Others took cues from Lorraine about how she felt about herself, and so she became the butt of jokes, which made her feel worse.

In ADHD-friendly therapy, Lorraine recognized this pattern and explored new ways of responding. Lorraine would visualize a party scene and imagine resetting her automatic response, so that the next time she went to a party she was prepared when she inevitably dropped food. Sure enough, the next time this happened Lorraine was able to laugh good-naturedly, pick up the food, and go back to engaging in conversation smoothly. Lorraine realized that the people she was talking to cared much more about discussing her talents as a teacher and her patient work with children than anything she was dropping!

When Lorraine took a step back to pause, reconsider her previously limited narrative, and take a whole-person perspective of herself, she was able to affirm herself in a way that was more accurate and helpful. "I bump into things and drop things—and it is also true that people don't even seem to notice—especially because I was helping them with their children's problems." Lorraine's view of herself had become more whole.

Moving into Wholeness

Many of us have grown up thinking we are either smart or dumb, organized or a mess, happy or sad, nice or mean. Or maybe we think that today we are good, tomorrow morning we switch over to bad, and then maybe in the afternoon we switch back over to good. Thinking in terms of drastic polarities like this keeps us flip-flopping from day to day and relegated to a space of reactivity instead of intentional thought and action. This leaves us with an unanchored narrative about who we are as individuals—who also happen to be women with ADHD. We can learn to rewrite the stories we tell ourselves about our lives, and we can separate ourselves from the identification with challenges we face (White and Epston 1990).

Healing means to "restore to wholeness." In order to heal, we need to be able to hold all of who we are in one whole image that embraces a widely diverse set of characteristics. That means no longer overfocusing on just our challenges or only on our strengths. Each of us

> *In order to heal, we need to be able to hold all of who we are in one whole image that embraces a widely diverse set of characteristics. That means no longer overfocusing on just our challenges or only on our strengths. Each of us is a complex human being.*

is a complex human being. When you remember that we are all imperfect, you will be able to move into a whole narrative with greater ease.

We all have changing perspectives, varying moods, periods of irrationality, and other times of clarity. Sometimes we yell at someone we love and we feel bad, and other times we are heartbreakingly kind to a stranger. We are many things at different times, even within the course of a single day. This complexity increases with an ADHD brain that fluctuates and reacts according to the conditions it is operating in at any given time.

When we use black and white, either/or, dichotomous thinking by overemphasizing one aspect of ourselves and dismissing the rest, we are engaging in *reductionism*, which is defined as the practice of simplifying a complex idea to the point of minimizing or distorting it. We literally reduce ourselves to one oversimplified or exaggerated attribute—typically our ADHD challenges. Moving into a more complete, whole narrative requires that we distance from reductionism and make room for a more expansive narrative. Opening up your view to encompass more of you, not less, will help you see yourself (ADHD and all) in a more balanced perspective.

Filling in Your Whole Picture

You may see your challenges with ADHD very clearly. In fact, you've probably overfocused on them forever. But there are likely some spots that you are blind to or that are difficult to access. So let's fill in the picture of you—meaning, give equal focus to your strengths or dreams or personal attributes that reflect your worth and value.

Reflection: **Moving Closer to Wholeness**

Below are several prompts to help you reflect upon and assess various aspects of your life with ADHD, including your strengths, challenges, personal attributes, and values. Read through the questions and write down anything that comes to mind.

Strengths

What are your zones of competency? What do you do really well that seems to come naturally?

_____

_____

_____

What could you teach or contribute to others?

_____

_____

_____

What skills or talents have you developed over the years?

_____

_____

_____

ADHD Challenges

What are your most challenging ADHD symptoms?

_____

_____

_____

Describe the issues you confront in daily life or in moving forward because of these challenges.

_____

_____

_____

_____

Realistically speaking, how might ADHD continue to show up in your life, even with medication and the right supports and tools?

_____

_____

_____

Personal Attributes

What makes you, you?

_____

_____

_____

How do you respond to the ups and downs of life at your best?

_____

_____

_____

What endures within you that makes the difference for you?

_____

_____

_____

What do you most appreciate about yourself?

_____

_____

_____

How would you describe yourself if you were a character in a book?

_____

_____

_____

What special qualities have you always had that you still embody (perseverance, determination, sense of humor, a fresh perspective, persistence, kindness, sensitivity, caring, compassion, hard work, creativity, originality, etc.)?

_____

_____

_____

_____

Creating an Authentic Path to Your Future

We often leave out experiences or information that doesn't fit with the incomplete picture or story we have been telling ourselves. If we only see the challenges, we won't have anywhere to add new positive experiences—and they will disappear before they have room to take root and grow. Oftentimes, we don't even know that we are missing the big picture.

After all, we can't see the picture when we're in the frame!

In order to begin living a new narrative and vision for your life, it's imperative that you practice pausing and staying in the freeze frame long enough to take in new information. This pause is absolutely essential for ADHD brains, as challenges with inhibition (putting on the brakes) make it difficult for the ADHD brain to slow down thoughts, reactions, and behaviors. Pausing helps you step out of the ADHD mind long enough to listen to what your core self has to say.

🪷 _Jamie's Story:_ The Whole Picture

When Jamie was occasionally a few minutes late for meetings at work, she would say to herself, "I'm a total screw-up! I can't do anything right! I'm an irresponsible, bad colleague." She would hold this mind-set during entire meetings. Jamie would be so preoccupied with worry that her coworkers were judging her that she would be unable to take in any information, even positive feedback. When Jamie's colleagues gave her good feedback, she would bat away their kind remarks by saying to herself, "They don't really mean it. I'm too much of a mess to do good work. They're just being polite."

As a result of working with a supportive therapist, Jamie began to shift her automatic negative responses. She began to say to herself, "I often run late with my projects and can keep working on that, but being late isn't my whole story. It doesn't define me or the quality of my *ideas. I sometimes have difficulty making myself understood, but that doesn't mean my ideas are bad." She began to notice more accurately what was really happening in these situations. "Actually, when I have a good idea, most people think it's amazing even if they don't understand it completely the first time I present it. I always bring a fresh perspective."*

Jamie began to notice when others gave her positive feedback, and she started to feel more confident and open. When she stopped letting her difficulties wipe out her ability to acknowledge her successes, Jamie actually began to build on them. In time, Jamie was able to give a more complete story about herself!

Personal Mission: Shaped by Values

We talk about the importance of values a lot but rarely stop and think about them as a guide that can help support ADHD. For women who are buffeted by the push and pull of the ADHD brain, it is critical to be able to return to an internal compass, or what some people call a *north star*, to know what we want our lives to be about. When we are feeling as if we are going in circles, it's helpful to pause and remind ourselves who and what is important to us. As an ADHD strategy, it can be helpful to create a cheat sheet to help us keep our values in mind.

For example, when we are pulled in many directions and by many competing thoughts, we may use our values to guide us to choose what is most important. From an ADHD perspective, it is often very difficult to sort this out, to bring to the foreground what is most important at a particular time. Locating a place inside us that kindly reminds us of our core values can break the feeling of overwhelm and overload many women with ADHD feel when pulled in many directions at once, both by their attention and their emotions.

For example, when you are confronted by needs from many people at once and feel confused as to which to respond to first, you might ask yourself: *What are my values that can guide my actions?*

- ☐ To be kind and empathic?
- ☐ To teach others to be responsible?
- ☐ To teach others to value differences?
- ☐ To teach others to follow rules?

Knowing our priorities in advance will give us a touchstone that we can refer to when we feel lost or drifting from our truths. This helps both from an ADHD perspective and in moving toward a meaningful life. By following our internal compass, our values—rather than the distractions caused by the ADHD mind—will guide our choices. When stuck in ADHD distractibility

("Oh, there's someone who needs me! I'll go in that direction." "Look! This is an interesting notice about an event, I'll go do that!"), we can easily confuse, dismiss, or derail our priorities, leaving us without energy or resources for the things that are most important to us. When we pause, we are able to make a more intentional decision that is more closely aligned with our mission, vision, and future goals.

An inner compass can take the form of a daily simple question: *Are my choices consistent with what I value?* This question will help center you and move you toward a future where you feel more whole. It will also help you decide what direction you need to take to manage ADHD at any given moment.

When you know what you value, you can write a personal mission statement, just like you would if you were running your own company. After all, you are running your own life! This can be a helpful shorthand (and ADHD-friendly) way to remember your values during triggered situations.

With ADHD, you likely get flooded or overwhelmed when your nervous system gets bombarded (Shaw et al. 2014). A cheat sheet can center you and help you keep acting out of your values when you are too tired or overwhelmed to think the situation through in the moment. For example, you might write your values and mission statement on a card and then post it near your desk, carry it in your wallet, or have it on your phone to serve as a quick reminder of your inner compass. Here's a sample:

> My mission is to be kind to others and to take the time to speak in respectful ways. I also expect and only accept respect in return. I want to help others in ways that I feel I am able to be helpful. I accept my limits in areas I am weaker in. I want to be kind but not intrusive. I want to be open and honest, especially when I feel it is important to discuss differences in my relationships.

Reflection: **Your Mission Statement**

To guide you toward authenticity as well as toward acting according to your core values, strengths, and challenges, answer the following questions. At the end, you will write your own mission statement

What is most meaningful to you?

_____

_____

_____

What do you want to stand for?

_____

_____

_____

What do you want your life to be about?

_____

_____

_____

What are your core values?

_____

_____

_____

What do you want people to know about you?

_____

_____

_____

When you look back on your life, what would you like to be able to say about yourself and your life?

_____

_____

_____

Try putting these details together in a few key points to summarize your personal mission.

_____

_____

_____

_____

_____

_____

Creating a Vision

In order to create a whole picture of your life and move into a more adaptive vision of your life, it helps to start by envisioning yourself living in a way that reflects these things. It's hard to work toward a more fulfilling future if you do not first have a feeling for what that lifestyle might look and feel like. Aim to be realistic about your ADHD challenges while also accounting for the other parts of you, such as your strengths and core values, as well as the possible supports that surround you.

Reflection: **Envisioning Exercise**

Doing this exercise helps you practice externalizing your ADHD challenges to create a bit of distance from your automatic thoughts and subsequent emotions. It provides the space necessary to make a judgment-free, intentional decision about how to live as successfully as possible with your ADHD challenges while enacting your personal values, aligning with your mission, and engaging in the world with a sense of purpose.

Grab a moment for yourself and take a few deep, cleansing breaths. Become as present in the moment as you can, letting go of your day up until and after this moment. Close your eyes and envision yourself waking up one, five, or ten years from now. Let yourself visualize as many details and sensory experiences as you can when imagining this scenario. Consider the following questions to guide your curiosity. Pause to write down or doodle some of the images as they come to mind, or return to them after you've spent some time immersed in your visualization.

What is the first thing you see around you?

How do you feel upon awakening?

How does your day unfold?

Which parts of your day feel good and authentic?

Which parts feel defeating or uncomfortable?

How are your actions reflective of your values and your mission during this day?

As you continue envisioning yourself going about your day, imagine yourself encountering ADHD moments or other personal or interpersonal barriers. When you encounter these moments, imagine yourself as someone who has grown and transformed in ways that feel good to you.

In the above scenario, which parts of you shine through that you are proud of? Which strengths bolster you?

Bring your vision to a close by imaging an ending to your day that feels complete and contented. What closing images or reflections come to mind?

When you can step back to consider the bigger picture, you can more easily witness all of the truths of yourself. For instance, if you are someone who tends to forget people's birthdays, instead of thinking of yourself as an awful person and terrible friend, you can take a step back to remember that you are a caring person who also has a knack for picking out awesome, meaningful gifts that have made many of your friends happy over the years. Gratitude and caring for others might be some of your personal values, and enacting those values might be part of your personal mission even if you do this in a nontraditional way.

When you see your whole self, you realize that it's actually not true that you are an awful person or a terrible friend. It is true, however, that you can be forgetful—a behavioral manifestation of the memory deficit caused by ADHD. Forgetfulness is a challenge, one that has likely had many consequences over the years. This is simply the truth. However, it is not the whole truth, and it certainly is not linked to your character, ability, or capacity to contribute to the world. Many other things are also true, and equally so. This is where you have a chance to shift your perspective.

As It Turns Out, Change Is Hard

Spoiler alert! We want to warn you that as soon as you start to think this wholeness and shining process could actually be fun, you might suddenly decide otherwise! Just as you feel on the brink of seeing a new way of doing this whole living-successfully-with-ADHD thing, you might surprisingly find yourself shutting down or encountering a strong feeling in your gut that makes you stop in your tracks.

Some women say that when they hit this point of "But I can't!," they experience a dizzy feeling. It's similar to when you go to the mall and find an array of overwhelming options and are blinded by the possibilities and beauty. The entire experience may feel too open, too unfamiliar, over- or under-stimulating, or even impossible. Without knowing why, you might find yourself going back to automatic thoughts such as, *Who am I kidding?* or *Whoops! Almost let myself fall into that trap of believing in something better.*

It helps if you expect to feel some barriers arise inside you: fears that you won't ever be able to do those things, doubts of your own abilities, conflicts about letting yourself dream and hope when you still have so many things you aren't doing, or those nagging expectations that you will disappoint yourself or others if you let yourself think too big or change too much.

As therapists, one of the hardest things about our work with women with ADHD is witnessing how easily they diminish themselves, shut down any budding belief in themselves, and fear trusting their ability to create a life that feels good and complete. One of the best things about our work with women with ADHD, on the other hand, is witnessing how strong, resilient, courageous, and determined they are when they set their sights on something wonderful and begin to let themselves believe again.

Recognizing Your Own Resistance

Truth be told, if you don't feel some anxiety about this you aren't letting yourself imagine! Starting off on a new path when it is unknown is always scary. When we open up old wounds, even if we have healed to some degree, we often still experience old aches in certain places and under particular conditions. Knowing that we are experiencing old wounds is the key to letting them exist—without responding to their compelling orders to stop our forward progress.

Resistance presents in various ways. For some, it is experienced as anxiety or fear. For others, it feels more like annoyance, frustration, or an inner pushing away of reminders or encouragement to do things differently. For yet others, resistance might manifest as feelings of sadness, loss, and helplessness that get in the way of active movement. Oftentimes, resistance catches us off guard, as it can be a deeply rooted, unconscious protection mechanism that automatically engages when we are faced with novel situations or stimuli.

🪷 *Michelle's Story:* Hitting a Wall of Resistance

When Sari and I began writing this book, I was filled with excitement, hope, and determination. Initially, I felt quite confident in my ability to do this. Pretty quickly, however, I became paralyzed. Not only was my ADHD brain struggling to get going and break through the organizational overwhelm of the process, but also anxiety and self-doubt seemed to keep creeping up.

I began to wonder if this book was as good of an idea as I first believed. I started disliking most of what I was able to write and worried that I wouldn't like the book in the end. I felt frustrated and doubtful. I even found myself not wanting to tell Sari that I was beginning to struggle, a kind of hiding compulsion. This seemed to be a pretty quick turnaround from my excitement just a week or so before. I thought, But I'm confident about this! Right? Why won't the words come? *So I did what women with ADHD often do: I fought harder to push through. I tried every ADHD support strategy and created the perfect environment in which to work. And still, I was stuck.*

When I sat down with Sari to discuss my hours of staring at a blank screen and blinking cursor, it became apparent that I was experiencing some resistance to taking this leap and putting myself out there more transparently. It is vulnerable to be a psychologist with my diagnosis writing a book for all to read, and then to hold myself accountable to walking the walk as well as I talk the talk.

Like you, ADHD still gets in my way, and I too have old doubts and fears that have long been unhelpful tagalongs on my journey. As ironic as it was, while writing this chapter, I was being deceptively sidelined by the very resistance and fear that I was trying to write about!

Sometimes feelings of resistance are obvious and telling, and other times they catch you off guard. When recognized, however, these sorts of inner barriers begin to give way to a greater belief in and commitment to intentional, empowered choices. Experiences of resistance, as frustrating and uncomfortable as they may be, are rich sources of information. When it comes to acts of desired, intentional change or taking calculated risks to live your best life, inner stop signs might actually mean "Go!"

Discovery: What's Your Brand of Resistance?

How do you experience inner resistance? Below are several examples of common experiences of inner barriers or blocks on the journey to shining more brightly. Check any that pertain to you so that you can more easily identify resistance when it arises.

For me, inner resistance to expanding my self in the world manifests as:

☐ Anxiety, feeling frozen, avoidance

☐ Irritation, annoyance, frustration

☐ Maximizing the obstacles and minimizing my abilities

☐ Self-doubt, self-criticism, immediately jumping to "I can't" or "I shouldn't"

☐ Giving up, isolating, shying away, hiding, convincing myself it doesn't matter

☐ Putting things off, "I will when _____" or "if…then" thinking

☐ Criticizing or dismissing others, particular situations, or certain stimuli

☐ Difficulty staying present and engaging fully

☐ Thinking of a million reasons why "I can't"

☐ Grief, loss, dwelling on the past

☐ Intense feelings of insecurity or vulnerability

☐ A sense of self-protection, withdrawal, becoming secretive, or hiding

☐ Other: _____

It is frightening to be on the brink of something you have always wanted, even for things such as love and success. You might feel afraid that it will all come crashing down around you. Let yourself notice when you feel most resistant to going forward. Those moments, those feelings, are information that will help you recognize where you might need to stretch.

Then, of course, there is another possibility: that things will go well. You might discover parts of yourself you always knew were there, buried under the paper and chaos. You may be afraid to look, to open up the door to the closet to begin the search. You may be afraid to find "it" and also afraid not to.

Resetting Your Default Settings

Like the preprogrammed settings on a computer that automatically kick in, all of us have behavioral and emotional defaults. Unless we know these behaviors and feelings are automatically operating, we won't react differently. That's why we have to go into our own emotional system preferences and recalibrate these automatic default responses to work in our favor.

Such automatic reactions often create resistance to considering a new vision for our lives and ourselves. This is especially confusing to our ADHD brains—we feel ready to move toward a more compelling future or fuller picture of ourselves, yet we also feel ourselves retreating.

🪷 *Sari's Story:* Preset Preferences

I remember the day when I discovered that there were preset preferences on my computer. Not only didn't I know how to change them, but I never knew they were operating! It wasn't until something was bothering me enough to investigate what was going on in the inner workings of the computer that I finally understood I had some control. I could go into my system preferences and reset these defaults to better conform to my true desires, the outcomes I wanted. I could decide! I didn't have free rein over my computer, and I had to work within the constraints of other realities, but I had a lot more control and choice than I previously knew.

Discovery: Change and ADHD

Below are some common default positions that many women assume they are stuck with. Imagine that you are about to make a change in your life. Or imagine that you just experienced an ADHD moment of blunder and you are feeling embarrassed and flustered.

Check off any of the sample assumptions that might be similar to your most common or comfortable default positions in such a scenario. Then circle one that you would like to work on reconfiguring (i.e., you will go into your own emotional system preferences and change them—just like on a computer!).

- ☐ I'll never be able to do anything differently or sustain positive change.

- ☐ I'll embarrass myself because of my difficult ADHD symptoms.

- ☐ I've tried opening up to others before and I ended up feeling misunderstood and judged. Why bother?

- ☐ It's never worked before. What will be any different this time?

- ☐ I won't be able to keep up or follow through.

- ☐ I can't tolerate the overwhelm this will cause.

- ☐ I'll give up after two weeks, per usual.

- ☐ I must be crazy to even let myself imagine something so good.

- ☐ I shouldn't need help. I have to push through all on my own.

- ☐ If it doesn't come easily or I make a mistake, then I should just give up.

- ☐ When things go wrong, it's my fault.

- ☐ I need to apologize for who I am.

- ☐ I knew this would happen. This is why I don't bother to try.

- ☐ If I had just used the strategy I learned, maybe I wouldn't be in this position, but clearly I'm even bad at having ADHD!

- ☐ ADHD is just an excuse. I know I'm really the problem.

Reflection: Which Defaults Do You Want to Reset?

Jot down or sketch a depiction of three current default settings.

Jot down or sketch a depiction of the default settings you would like to have instead.

When you remember who you are at the core, what you value, and your own worth—despite or even because of your unique challenges—you will be able to communicate from a place that honors all of who you are. You will be able to remember: "I have these strengths and challenges, and I am much more than that. I am all this and more." As David Giwerc, the founder of ADDCA, the largest ADHD coaches training organization, says in his book *Permission to Proceed*:

When you give yourself permission to proceed with your natural self, the one who is in integrity with who you are, and pay attention to the cherished values aligned with the spirit and passion of your heart, you make a transformational choice. Just by granting yourself permission to proceed, you set out on a path to picturing a world of possibilities and creating a powerful new reality! (2011, 241)

ADHD-Friendly Chapter Takeaways

🪷 Discovering who you are as a whole woman and where your authentic core sense of self wants to go sets you on the path to making more fulfilling choices about your life and relationships.

🪷 Resistance is inevitable—and something to embrace and work through. When you can accept that doubt, fear, and loss are natural responses to this kind of change, you can begin to let yourself hope again.

🪷 You can have fear and experience inner barriers to the change process and still begin to shine more brightly.

CHAPTER 7

Shine as You Are

Becoming Comfortable with Being Seen, Heard, and Known

In this chapter, we want you to become more comfortable revealing your strengths and letting yourself shine by taking small steps to reveal your unique gifts, personality, and interests. You will be encouraged to expand, to claim more space in your life, and to create a larger life. The goal is to work against your impulse to shrink back into smallness in the face of differences. You will learn ways to push gently past the edge of your comfort zone to reach for the vision you identified and explored throughout chapter 6.

When we use the word "shine" we aren't necessarily or specifically talking about performance, dominating a room, or a special achievement. Of course, if that's what you want and are ready, go for it! Our point is, however, that you don't need to think of shining in a professional or traditional sense. Instead, think of it in the sense of taking up more room in your life. Imagine letting yourself expand and feel entitled through your words or actions, making yourself more visible, significant, and equal. You deserve to be seen, heard, and known. You are worthy and capable of playing the main character in your life, even with your ADHD moments, trials, and tribulations.

Expanding

Women with ADHD are just as good and valuable as anyone else, though they often feel "less than" and shrink back from life as a result. Hopefully, at this point on your journey, through this new perspective and deep work, you have discovered that there are a great variety of situations in which you can expand instead of diminish yourself.

A Declaration of Independence for Women with ADHD

As women with ADHD, we have rights that are vulnerable to surrendering because of our difficulties and differences. Even though we have challenges, we need to recognize that we do not forfeit our right to a fulfilling life, equal relationships, and the pursuit of meaning and passion because of them.

> *Even though we have challenges, we need to recognize that we do not forfeit our right to a fulfilling life, equal relationships, and the pursuit of meaning and passion because of them.*

America's founding document, the Declaration of Independence, declares that we each are endowed with a set of freedoms that are our birthright. Below is a version of the Declaration of Independence for women with ADHD, revealing the rights that give us freedom from oppressive thoughts and patterns. (You can print a copy at http://www.newharbinger.com/32617.) Post it where you will see it frequently, so that you can continue to absorb its message and act in accordance with those rights.

Declaration of Independence
for Women with ADHD

- The right to have connection, even though you have challenges

- The right to pursue your talents, even though you have challenges

- The right to speak, reveal your ideas, and be known, even though you have differences

- The right to claim and pursue your hopes and dreams, even though you have challenges

- The right to take time and make space for yourself, even though you have challenges

- The right to live shame-free and be treated with respect, even though you are imperfect

- The right to ask for help, even though you have strengths

Expanding in Relationships

You have the right to have connection, even though you have challenges.

As a woman with ADHD, you likely have had many experiences during which you gradually learned to shrink back in relationships, give up power, or disconnect and avoid. It's time for you to expand within connection and feed the relationships that sustain you, without withdrawing or handing over your power. You have the right to have connection and closeness.

Many women with ADHD struggle with maintaining contact and closeness with friends and extended family. Relationship maintenance is difficult for women with ADHD because it involves consistent actions that are not as stimulating and engaging as one-on-one, face-to-face contact, and these actions often require strong executive functioning skills. If this is the case for you, it's likely that you care very deeply about other people, but your friends and family members may misinterpret ADHD symptoms or related behaviors to mean that you aren't invested in the relationship. Forgetting to say "Happy Birthday," becoming distracted on the phone, and responding to text messages or phone calls a week late are just a few examples of these frequently misunderstood behaviors.

You may find that you shrink back from closeness with friends and extended family because you feel misunderstood or afraid that you have disappointed others due to inconsistency in contact. The anxiety and avoidance that typically follow can take things to a higher level of interpersonal gridlock or isolation. You might find yourself distancing from, or even actively avoiding, people you once enjoyed because of this rising anxiety and shame. It's easy to see how what starts out as ADHD may turn into a relationship issue.

Expanding into deeper, more meaningful connections with people who value you as an equal involves taking the risk to reach out to them—perhaps *especially* to those you have been avoiding out of shame and fear. It might mean harnessing the courage to do the opposite of your habitual pull to hide, pretend, or isolate. You deserve to have connection even though you have challenges that might be difficult for some to understand. You also have the right to be treated with respect in the face of those moments.

Reflection: Expanding in Relationships

You have the right to have connection, even though you have challenges.

How have you been holding back this part of you?

_____

_____

_____

_____

How can you expand into connection this week?

_____

_____

_____

_____

Expanding Your Strengths

You have the right to pursue your talents, even though you have challenges.

You may have pulled back from developing or demonstrating your talents or interests over the years, feeling you would be criticized, be unable to follow through, or end up disappointing others.

When you consider taking action toward demonstrating your talents or expanding your interests, you might notice guilt crop up about having so many things left "undone." Another common fear is that putting yourself out there in this way would leave you way too exposed to failing, criticism, or disappointing yourself or others.

You might worry that others will judge you or reinforce your own self-criticism. You might hesitate to step into the spotlight, fearing that others will say things like, "She's always running late, and now she wants to take the time to try out for a local theater production?" Or "She can't return a phone call, but she just posted on social media about a new yoga class?"

Shining a light on your strengths and taking action to highlight what you're good at and passionate about involves taking the risk to confront these fears and voices—both within and without, real or imagined. You have the right to share your strengths and contribute to the world around you even though you struggle with symptoms of ADHD.

Reflection: Expanding Your Strengths

You have the right to pursue your talents, even though you have challenges.

How have you been holding back this part of you?

_____

_____

_____

_____

_____

How can you expand into your strengths and talents this week?

_____

_____

_____

_____

Expanding Your Voice

You have the right to speak, reveal your ideas, and be known, even though you have differences.

Expanding your voice is essential to letting yourself be known. It is understandably difficult to lean into the vulnerability necessary for others to get to know you. This kind of expansion involves taking the risk to state your needs, let yourself be noticed and known, and say something that reveals more of who you are in the face of differences. This can mean revealing what you have accomplished, created, thought about, hoped for, or dreamed about, along with your opinions, wishes, and idiosyncrasies.

We want to clarify that this does not mean you should tell everything to everyone, all the time. It means to expand, to reveal little bits here and there, like in the Hansel and Gretel fable, leaving clues of bread crumbs that may eventually lead people to who you are.

This way of expanding requires thinking about, choosing, and deciding to whom the various parts of you should be known. You have the right to have a voice, even though you have challenges.

❁ *Holly's Story:* Owning Her Strengths

Holly, a woman in her midthirties, gets together with a group of women from college a few times a year. At this point, all her friends are either getting married or having children. So while the others chatted about weddings, houses, and fertility at a recent gathering, Holly remained quiet. Her life was going in a distinctly different direction, not just because of her ADHD but because of her unusual level of success in her field.

Not only did Holly refrain from volunteering any information, but friends didn't ask about her life. She got the impression that the others were staying away from asking her questions about her life because it didn't involve the same things, as if they felt they didn't want to embarrass her. Ironically, Holly was by far the most accomplished professionally in the group. She had an advanced degree in science and was part of an exciting research team funded to find a cure for Alzheimer's disease.

Holly wondered how to handle this. Should she just volunteer information about her work? Should she listen good-naturedly to them and let the hours just go by exchanging pleasantries?

Holly realized that her sensitivity to differences in this situation wasn't about her ADHD or her difficulties; in fact, it was about her strengths! The truth was that Holly was happy with her choices. It was only when confronted with her differences and unmet gender role expectations that she wasn't sure how to communicate in a way that put herself back in the equation. Gender taboos she had internalized about appearing to brag or seem better than others were playing a role as well.

When Holly felt more sure of her power to give voice to her differences, the next time she was together with these friends she decided to reveal the life she valued and claim her right to be known. She didn't cut off relationships and she didn't retreat. Instead, Holly helped her friends understand by approaching the idea of differences directly instead of minimizing or defending them. She said, "I want you to know I am different in that I don't want to have children. My legacy is going to be about my work, which is very exciting to me. I would love to tell you about what I'm working on!"

Reflection: Expanding Your Voice

You have the right to speak, reveal your ideas, and be known, even though you have differences.

How have you been holding back this part of you?

_____

_____

_____

_____

_____

Write down ways you can expand into using your voice this week.

_____

_____

_____

_____

Expanding Your Dreams

You have the right to claim and pursue your hopes and dreams, even though you have challenges.

Due to your challenges, you may feel as if you must give up your dreams because you don't deserve to have them. This may cause you a great deal of longing, yearning, pain, and sadness. Not only may you regret your unfulfilled dreams, but you may also feel consigned to a class of unworthy people condemned to some kind of organizational purgatory, doomed forever to go through piles of paper, boxes, and undone tasks. You may feel sentenced to forced labor for eternity and robbed of your birthright that everyone shares: to hope and dream, despite any difficulties, human flaws, or disorganization. Because ADHD is a lifelong struggle, you can't put your life on hold. Instead, you can claim your right to your hopes and dreams while you slowly work on these other areas of challenges.

This kind of expansion involves taking the risk to envision and move toward a life of purpose and meaning, even though much remains disorganized or unfinished. Claiming your right to hopes and dreams means enlarging and making visible what you have created or envisioned.

Reflection: Expanding Your Dreams

You have the right to claim and pursue your hopes and dreams, even though you have challenges.

How have you been holding back this part of you?

_____

_____

_____

_____

How can you expand into your dreams this week?

_____

_____

_____

_____

Expanding Your Personal Space

You have the right to take time and make space for yourself, even though you have challenges.

We encourage you to enlarge and enhance your own life instead of waiting until everyone else is taken care of. This includes taking time for self-care, relaxation, and pleasure instead of over-working to cover up your ADHD challenges. Depletion is the opposite of expansion.

Expanding in this sense means that you have the right to put yourself and your needs (your health!) first at times, instead of reflexively putting everyone else's needs in front or in place of yours. Remember, you can't pour from an empty cup! Give yourself permission to take time for yourself to play purely for the sake of having fun. At the very least, it means don't schedule yourself out of your own to-do list!

> **Depletion is the opposite of expansion.**

This kind of expansion involves claiming and taking up more space in the actual room interpersonally as well as inside yourself. When you allow yourself the right to take space for yourself, you claim your worth and deserved place in the world. You are deserving of this, even with your challenges.

❈ *Amber's Story:* Claiming Her Space

Amber had spent every weekend at her girlfriend Miranda's apartment for months. The relationship was progressing beautifully, but ADHD was creating some annoyances.

Going to Miranda's for the weekend meant packing an overnight bag and planning several logistical steps in advance. The transition back into her routine at home posed predictable obstacles that Amber couldn't get used to. The small things were becoming big hurdles.

Nearly every weekend, Amber forgot to pack something. One weekend she left her meds at home, another she forgot her toothbrush, another she forgot her computer charger, and on and on. Every time Amber packed up to leave Miranda's, she secretly longed to leave some things behind, things she wouldn't have to keep repacking over and over. The two had already agreed that Amber would move in when her own lease was up, but as close as she came to asking to leave a few things at Miranda's, she shied away as a million doubts and questions came up.

"What if she feels bothered by my clutter? What if I seem too confident or comfortable? What if I take up too much space?"

Amber felt both fear and a sense of inner resistance to letting her guard down and letting comfort in. She was literally and figuratively afraid to take up space, and she anticipated judgment and rejection, despite any indication that she was anything but adored and accepted by her partner. Amber acknowledged that she sometimes felt that having someone accept her so unconditionally and not reinforce old stories about her ADHD challenges felt a bit too good to be true.

After processing this conundrum in therapy and spending time with an encouraging friend, Amber began to think more clearly about what she really wanted and needed. She did some journaling and even took notes on her phone whenever something triggered her old fears and barriers to asserting her true desires. She paid careful attention to signs that Miranda did indeed love and accept her fully, and she recorded those too to keep them close in her memory. Instead of confirming her worst fears, Amber saw more and more evidence that Miranda wanted her to take up more space, not less! Amber realized that beneath these fears and old stories, she actually felt strongly that she was a valuable partner and entitled to equal space.

Once Amber felt clearer about what she wanted and needed, she decided on a simple and direct way to get to the heart of what she really wanted to know. Over dinner one night, Amber spoke up: "I'd like to leave a few things here, like shampoo and my toothbrush. How do you feel about that?" Amber didn't prolong the request or talk around it, she simply inquired about what she most wanted to know. Miranda responded with a playful laugh and said, "Of course! I want you to be here…and to have fresh breath!" Amber found her way to the heart of the matter and claimed her space, within her environment and relationship, with just one question.

Reflection: Expanding Your Personal Space

You have the right to take time and make space for yourself, even though you have challenges.

How have you been holding back this part of you?

_____

_____

_____

_____

_____

How can you expand your personal space this week?

_____

_____

_____

_____

Expanding Your Self-Worth

You have the right to live shame-free and be treated with respect, even though you are imperfect.

You have to come to terms with your own worth. You do not forfeit the right to be treated with respect even when you have difficulties.

You have a right to walk away from toxic help. By toxic help, we mean support or attempts at helping that come along with harmful doses of criticism. One example might be a friend helping to organize a room in your home and immediately commenting, "How can you live like this?!" Toxic help isn't help at all.

> **You are not indebted to others because you have ADHD.**

Even when someone has done a great deal to help you, you have the right to express disappointment, frustration, or anger. You and others can express feelings or grievances in a respectful way. You are not indebted to others because you have ADHD.

This kind of expansion involves taking the risk to express your feelings even though you need help. You have the right to live without the confines of shame and be treated with respect, even though you are imperfect.

Reflection: **Expanding Your Self-Worth**

You have the right to live shame-free and be treated with respect, even though you are imperfect.

How have you been holding back this part of you?

_____

_____

_____

_____

How can you expand your sense of self-worth this week?

_____

_____

_____

_____

Expanding Your Support

You have the right to ask for help, even though you also have strengths.

If you are like many women with ADHD, you might pass for "normal" so well that people don't realize you are covering up difficulties. There is also the possibility, in this case, that you have set up your life in a way that allows you to use your strengths, and that compensates for your challenges. This is not pretending. This happens when you have been able to create situations or put yourself in environments in which you can flourish and succeed. You may feel like an imposter because only you know the disorganization or the hard work and compensation behind the scenes.

It is important to remember this: you are not an imposter in these situations. You are someone who has found a way to use her strengths. They are real. You are not fooling anyone who sees your real strengths. You need to own both sides—strengths and challenges—as a whole person. Neither side defines you or cancels out the other part. You can be smart, talented, and successful in some areas, and you can still have struggles and let yourself ask for help when you need it.

This kind of expansion involves taking the risk to ask for what you need even though people might not know you are struggling. Even though you have strengths and might pass as neurotypical, you still have the right to ask for help and support.

Reflection: Expanding Your Support

You have the right to ask for help, even though you also have strengths.

How have you been holding back this part of you?

_____

_____

_____

_____

_____

How can you expand your support system this week?

_____

_____

_____

_____

Stepping Stones: Identifying the Edge of Your Comfort Zone

The concept of a comfort zone is something most people can easily identify in themselves. One way to think about it is an internal state where things feel familiar, where you feel at ease and able to easily meet the demands of your environment and experience low levels of stress.

You may be thinking, *Feeling calm and in control sounds like a good place to be when making a change or taking a new action to expand myself. It's good to be stress-free, right?* Well, to a certain extent, yes, of course—within reason. This is what psychologist Daniel Goleman says:

When demands become too great for us to handle, when the pressure overwhelms us, too much to do with too little time or support, we enter the zone of bad stress. Just beyond the optimal zone at the top of the performance arc, there is a tipping point where the brain secretes too many stress hormones, and they start to interfere with our ability to work well, to learn, to innovate, to listen, and to plan effectively. (2012)

Finding the Sweet Spot

The key to finding your "optimal performance zone" (White 2009)—to stepping into a new way of doing things—is to find the right amount and kind of stress. This is a state where you are not overloaded but not understimulated either. Locate the place where you can keep the fire lit and the embers smoldering, without burning down the house! Or, as author and speaker Neale Donald Walsch (2012) puts it: "Life begins at the end of your comfort zone."

Notice that you're being invited to lean into some degree of stress, not shy away from it. As psychologist Abraham Maslow is reported to have said, "One can choose to go back toward safety or forward toward growth. Growth must be chosen again and again; fear must be overcome again and again." Personal growth doesn't emerge from a comfortable space; creation is messy, and discomfort accompanies everything worth birthing. When you remember this, you will be erecting the internal scaffolding on which to build future confidence and successes.

Expanding beyond your comfort zone takes courage and practice. It isn't something that just happens—you have to work at it, sometimes moving two steps ahead only to fall back one. This is how change happens. Instead of falling into the trap of all-or-nothing thinking, which so often derails and defeats, you can generate alternatives to bringing your stress to an optimal level, without retreating and discarding all possibilities.

> *Personal growth doesn't emerge from a comfortable space; creation is messy, and discomfort accompanies everything worth birthing.*

You Are Capable

Moving out of your comfort zone requires an inner sense of capability. Instead of perceiving experiences as happening to you—as out of your control and in the hands of other people and circumstances—retrieve your sense of personal power and recognize that you have influence over what happens next. This is called developing an *internal locus of control*. Your choices matter!

Research has shown that people who have a greater internal locus of control generally feel better about themselves, are more proactive, cope with adversity more effectively, and experience less anxiety and depression. The challenge, however, is that our sense of internal versus external locus of control can easily change based on our daily experiences of success or failure (Ryon and Gleason 2014). As a person with ADHD, you may have experienced what you consider to be many false starts. As a result, you may have come to believe that steps you take toward your goals won't matter or make a difference. As you learn to view the changes you want to make as intentional choices under your control, you will gradually find it easier to stretch toward growth and expansion. This comes as a result of making small decisions that lead you to new experiences of success.

🪷 *Janna's Story:* Going Big by Starting Small

Janna knew that an important part of her vision for a more expanded sense of herself was to become more involved in yoga. Her vision was to join some kind of yoga community or training program.

When Janna found a retreat that was exactly what she had imagined for herself, she felt very excited. After a few moments, though, she felt surprised as she noticed fear and discomfort setting in. She had found the actual experience that she had dreamed of—a yoga retreat in a beautiful part of the world with a community of like-minded people and expert trainers—yet, when it came time to register, she found she was not following through. It didn't make sense to her.

As a result of the untangling process, Janna was able to figure out which part of this inaction was a result of her ADHD and which part was from the anxiety of moving out of her comfort zone. She was also able to recognize when she started to fall into her default position of berating herself for not jumping in full steam ahead.

Janna realized that she was not going to motivate herself by being mean to herself. Janna remembered that she could be an active agent in making her dream happen; instead of jumping in headfirst, she could start with a small, simple push out of her comfort zone. She didn't have to take the full plunge right away.

Janna decided she needed to inch toward her goal instead of pushing so hard. She found a local yoga workshop and asked a friend to text her a gentle reminder about signing up.

Though Janna's friend texted her, as promised, Janna still resisted taking the final action of signing up. Janna realized she was just too anxious to do this on her own. Instead of giving up, though, Janna had her friend come over and sit with her at the computer for moral support. Finally, with this extra emotional support that quieted her anxiety, Janna followed through and signed up for the workshop. From an ADHD perspective, arranging for her friend to come over served as a "go" button (a great ADHD strategy), creating the actual time and energy to take this action.

After a successful experience at the local workshop, Janna felt comfortable signing up for an ongoing class in the same yoga method. She eventually became friendly with a classmate who also wanted to attend the out-of-town retreat that Janna had originally discovered. The next year when the workshop was offered again, Janna's comfort zone edge had expanded, and it was right at the spot that allowed her without hesitation to sign up and attend.

When you come across a way to shine or encounter an experience that would give you a chance to be seen, heard, or known—or to fulfill your vision and new narrative—you might find yourself feeling discomfort and resistance. If so, take note of it. Experiencing discomfort might mean that you are right at the edge of your comfort zone and, if you keep gently exploring, you might push through the resistance and into new, exciting territory.

If, as you move increasingly toward the edge of your comfort zone, you find that your hesitation and anxiety persist, it might be a sign that you need to back up one step and try something smaller. Instead of thinking about everything that needs to be done, think in terms of taking the *next* and *smallest* step toward your goal. If you are still feeling overwhelmed or confused, break it down further to an even smaller step.

> *Experiencing discomfort might mean that you are right at the edge of your comfort zone and, if you keep gently exploring, you might push through the resistance and into new, exciting territory.*

The point is to neither retreat completely and give up nor push through to a step too big. Like Janna, you might need human support to help you select a time and an action that will move you forward as you take a new risk.

Finding Your Edge

At some point, your comfort zone and your vision will begin to slowly overlap. This will take time. If you keep taking your smallest next step—and continue moving in your desired direction—you will get there!

Reflection: **Your Comfort Zone**

What step at the edge of your comfort zone can you identify to help you move in the direction of your vision?

_____

_____

_____

_____

_____

_____

ADHD-Specific Comfort Zones

In the same way that you need to increase your comfort zone for your vision, you might want or need to expand your comfort zone in ADHD-specific situations.

For example, your goal may be to learn more about ADHD and get emotional support and practical strategies. In this situation, you may feel comfortable enough to watch a webinar but not ready enough to reach out to a coach or an organizer. On the other hand, you may feel ready to go to a local support group or even contact a coach. At some point you may feel ready to take the more risky action of going to a national ADHD conference out of town.

Discovery: Moving Toward the Edge of Your ADHD Comfort Zone

Here are examples of how and where women with ADHD often want to challenge themselves to move toward the edge of their ADHD comfort zone. Check any that resonate with you.

☐ Asking for accommodations at work

☐ Asking for changes at home

☐ Asserting ADHD needs to others without disclosing a diagnosis

☐ Asking loved ones to learn more about ADHD

☐ Prioritizing time for myself and keeping that commitment

☐ Trying something new and sticking to it a bit longer than before

☐ Meeting new people, going to support groups

☐ Making phone calls

☐ Rebuilding friendships after losing touch

☐ Going back to school, getting a certificate, taking a class for fun

☐ Asserting myself with loved ones

☐ Getting more involved with ADHD help and education

☐ Helping other women with ADHD

☐ Volunteering to help an ADHD organization or awareness event

Reflection: Where Is Your Edge?

Describe where, in your own life with ADHD, you would like to stretch yourself. What sorts of behaviors do you engage in within your comfort zone?

_____

_____

_____

_____

_____

How do you feel and interact with yourself and others there?

_____

_____

_____

_____

_____

What step toward the edge are you ready to take this week?

_____

_____

_____

_____

As you move forward in your journey to be seen, heard, and known, you can continually refer back to and actively engage with the Declaration of Independence for Women with ADHD that presents seven rights to claim for yourself, even though you have challenges. You are in the process of creating a larger life; you have the right to claim it!

ADHD-Friendly Chapter Takeaways

🪷 In order to become comfortable with expanding your sense of self, your life, and your relationships, remember that you have rights—even though you have challenges.

🪷 You have value, even though you have challenges. And you can ask for help, even though you have strengths.

🪷 Become comfortable with expanding yourself and claiming your rights, even if that means going slowly, small step by small step, toward your dreams.

PART III

Bolder

"Life loves to be taken by the lapel and told: 'I'm with you, kid. Let's go.'"

—Maya Angelou

Part III of this workbook, Bolder, focuses on taking action to step into our life with gusto and intention as women with ADHD. As Angelou is quoted as saying, life requires—and is worth—our active engagement. Leaning into our unique, complicated lives with an attitude of willingness and an openness to experience are what move living into being richly, authentically alive.

There is an additional, crucial consideration that must be part of the equation for whole-life living for women with ADHD. The truth is that, for us, more time, effort, support, and resilience are required to create the space to lean in and engage with life more actively. While it is more work to do this, the upshot is that, because we *need* to do it, we can't take it for granted or depend on chance.

That means we have the great possibility of living and choosing a full, open life, one that doesn't happen just by accident. When we achieve it, it is because we have claimed it and earned it, every difficult step of the way! When we own it, integrate it, and feel proud of it, we can call on this resilience during difficult periods of our lives. What a great feeling of security, ironically, that hard work can provide.

What are you waiting for? Step forward, boldly!

CHAPTER 8

Take Center Stage

Commanding Attention

Leading a bold life as a woman with ADHD involves becoming increasingly visible, speaking with a stronger voice, and taking and holding the attention of other people. In doing so, you enable yourself to step more fully into a rich, authentic life full of confidence and clarity. We now explore how you can begin to live increasingly on the center stage of your own life.

Taking Center Stage

It might feel uncomfortable, at first, for you to read the words "take center stage." You might feel awkward saying those words out loud because you worry about coming across as conceited or self-centered. Whatever your immediate reaction, notice it and take it in stride; many of us need some time to cozy up to the idea that we can command attention and still, at the very same time, remain humble, connected, and accepted.

Taking center stage doesn't mean being narcissistic or that everything should revolve around you. It means acting in ways that keep you relevant, equal, and participating in reciprocal relationships. It's not about showing off, but it *is* about participating fully and equally in life.

Center stage can represent many things to you or take a wide variety of forms depending on your particular goals, needs, and dreams. This can cover a big range of situations. Here are a few examples:

- Being willing to "bother" people more with your own needs and wants, decreasing how much you accommodate everyone else

- Performing or presenting in front of people to reveal a talent, interest, or your ideas

- Prioritizing your needs and self-care in spite of other demands for your care and attention

- Letting people know you have something of value to say or something that is important to you that you want to share

You're Worth a Seat at the Table

Holding attention may feel unfamiliar to you. If you have inattentive ADHD, you may be more familiar with living in the background or being overlooked. If you are more extroverted or someone with the combined-presentation type of ADHD, you may talk or move around more, but you may still have experienced the wound of being disregarded.

In either case, you may not have had a lot of experience taking the attention and holding it in a powerful or direct way. Perhaps due to your ADHD or your beliefs about yourself (i.e., tangles), you may have gotten in the practice of transmitting—verbally or nonverbally, consciously or unconsciously—that you neither believe in nor value what you have to share.

Being bold and having presence doesn't mean you have to share your accomplishments. Instead, it's about deeply believing that when you are with other people, whether you are quiet or more hyperactive, you deserve a place at the table or in the group, whatever the situation.

But Why Is It So hard?

Women with ADHD can struggle with verbal expression in various ways, which very directly creates a barrier to being seen, known, and heard. Difficulty organizing our thoughts, holding the thread of a story for several minutes, remembering where we are in a conversation, and not going off on rabbit trails can cause anxiety for those of us who want to take center stage at work or in our personal life.

Here's a story that demonstrates the steady small steps of holding the spotlight of other people's attention a little longer than you may be comfortable with. This has to do with the boost that the right medication can give you to deal with the actual ADHD. Lots of people take medication and get the fuel, but not everyone learns to take it for a ride.

🪷 *Sari's Story:* Taking the Stage

The first time I took medication for ADHD was also the first time I told a whole story at dinner to a group of people. The amazing thing was, to my great surprise, people listened! This was an example of ADHD medication serving as a foundation, giving me the actual fuel and mental organization to string that many words together in an understandable way and sustain that for at least five minutes! That was a record for me at that time in this kind of situation. In other words, there was no rehearsal, no script, just me and my brain on full display!

I took a deep breath and dove in. The words came out in order, and I held the stage of the dinner party for five minutes longer than I had ever before. I was just telling a little story about something of little significance that had happened that I found interesting, but it required a lot of mental organization to tell the story in a way that was understandable, chronological, and compelled others' attention. It also required that I overcome fears that they would drift off from boredom or that I would give up, embarrassingly unable to really convey what I wanted. The actual story I told was inconsequential, but the risk of extending myself more onto center stage at that moment and finding my voice was huge; it stretched my comfort zone to make me ready for a bigger step next time.

With diagnosis and then medication, I had access to my thoughts in a new way. I now had the fuel to sustain my thoughts, but then I had to take the risk. The medication gave me the brain conditions that made that possible, but it was me, Sari, who took the risk. I had to believe that I had something interesting to say—and that it would be okay if no one else thought the same.

If you are an inattentive woman who often has trouble even beginning to speak, this story might have resonated with you. While women on the hyperactive and impulsive side of the ADHD spectrum might not identify fully with speechlessness, they also experience barriers around communication.

While the quieter kind of woman with ADHD holds back, others—often with combined presentation—might dive in impulsively and talk a great deal. If you identify with the less verbally inhibited brand of ADHD, you may find you talk about many subjects, connecting one idea to another without a pause. You might become frustrated with yourself for not holding back more in your speech despite your best intentions.

In these cases, the listener might feel bombarded, lost, confused, annoyed, taken aback, or even hurt by an onslaught of words or a statement that slipped through your filter seemingly out of nowhere. That person might not have a chance to contribute to or end the conversation, leading to feelings of being stuck or of being unequal partners in the interaction. Sometimes words serve as defenses; they can form walls that keep others out instead of building bridges to connection. You, too, may feel invisible.

On the other hand, if you find that you talk too fast, too much, or in too circular a fashion, you may need to learn to slow things down, take time to pause, and make a few written or mental notes. Instead of diving in, you may need to proceed more cautiously, dipping one toe in first. You may need to learn to observe the situation and the interactions that are going on. You may need to pause and think about what impact you want to make before jumping in.

Whichever category you fall into, the goal is the same: to make an impact, to be seen, heard, and known. You will need to take the risk of being uncomfortable and vulnerable when trying new ways of opening up. While medication can help women with ADHD speech patterns to pause, focus, and organize their thoughts to facilitate communication, presence and practice are the best ways to get used to expressing yourself in a new way. With this approach, you can begin to notice what you need to do to let people know what you have inside.

> *Taking your place in the world starts with what you believe about your right to be here.*

As you begin to expand how you speak to others, remember that it's not merely about how much you talk or how much time you take up. It's about intention, presence, and connection.

People take their cues from you. Taking your place in the world starts with what you believe about your right to be here. Believe that you're worth a seat at the table.

Three Ways to Stay in the Spotlight

Some challenges you face are the result of being a woman, and others are because of your ADHD. The combination of ADHD and the cultural messages or lessons you have learned as a woman can be a powerful mixture that lead you to be overaccommodating to others, to be less direct when speaking about your own ideas or needs, and to retreat from being seen clearly. Conversely, here are three main ways to stay in the spotlight of your life:

- Be less accommodating

- Use your voice

- Become more visible

Be Less Accommodating

One way to stay in the center of the stage is to decrease how much you revolve around the needs of others. (Even writing this feels heretical, so let us explain.)

Have you learned to accommodate others and push your own needs away, instead of asking for the help you need and deserve? As a woman with ADHD, you probably need accommodations or support to function optimally, but you might also find yourself shying away from asserting this while you continue to put others first. You might accommodate in an effort to stop the overload of other people's needs and demands and emotions, to reduce your stress in the short run, or because it's simply what you learned about your role in a family or group early on in life. If you have established an identity as a caretaker or derive self-worth from being needed, you are very likely to put yourself on the back burner, which can ultimately scorch your health and sense of self over time. Overaccommodating is a sign that you are moving off the center stage of your own life.

With ADHD, you may be easily drawn to shiny objects. This can include people who occupy a lot of space in your life or need your help, or situations where you can comfortably take a supportive or secondary role. But you don't always have to be in a supporting role.

> *Overaccommodating is a sign you are moving off the center stage of your own life.*

What are some actions you can take to be a major player in your life?

- ☐ Asking others for help

- ☐ Making my own needs known

- ☐ Setting the agenda and letting others orbit around me sometimes

- ☐ Letting myself be the focus of attention longer than typical for me

- ☐ Claiming time, space, and care for myself

- ☐ Sharing my opinions, ideas, or skills more assertively

- ☐ Other: _____

In benign or low-stakes situations, we encourage you to find opportunities to practice creating and tolerating a slight discomfort in other people, so that you can increase the time you allow yourself to say what you want or need. This reversal in your approach—toward an empowered perspective instead of a disempowered place of perpetual stuckness—will help you feel more prepared to ask for what you need or to share more of yourself in any scenario.

Use Your Voice

Many women struggle to find and use their voice. When cultural and gender barriers combine with ADHD challenges, women face a complex intersection of blockades that can shut out their voice and render them speechless. As you traverse the terrain of self-expansion and empowerment as a woman with ADHD, you will benefit from examining how you can use your voice to take and hold the attention of others in order to make an impact.

In our concept of boldness, speaking becomes easier when you believe in and understand your vision. Harnessing your voice requires that you rewrite *any* narrative you have created that undermines it, and then claim your right to speak up and be heard, both alone and with others. Audre Lorde's (1977) quote below speaks to the inner playfulness and creative spirit of many women with ADHD who want to be themselves and lead a full and meaningful life with their uniqueness, not without or in spite of it.

> And the speaking will get easier and easier. And you will find you have fallen in love with your own vision, which you may never have realized you had. And you will lose some friends and lovers, and realize you don't miss them. And new ones will find you and cherish you. And you will still flirt and paint your nails, dress up and party, because, as I think Emma Goldman said, "If I can't dance, I don't want to be part of your revolution." And at last you'll know with surpassing certainty that only one thing is more frightening than speaking your truth. And that is not speaking.

Using your voice is powerful! Your voice can impact other people, empower yourself, and facilitate change. It can uplift, it can deflate, it can assert, it can wound, and it can heal. The more you practice owning and expressing your voice—using it with intention, confidence, and care— the more you will experience a feeling of power. We don't mean power over other people but rather power that comes from within and conveys a quiet, confident sort of assuredness that only comes with a feeling of being at peace with yourself, without apology.

Effective communication very rarely comes naturally to anyone, ADHD or not. It is a skill that deserves time, presence, and cultivation. Remember, we don't speak for the sake of speaking; we speak to connect.

HOW AND WHY WE SELF-SILENCE

Many women (not just women with ADHD) use qualifiers or minimizers to soften the impact of their communication when, in reality, their true desire is to increase their impact. This is especially likely to happen when they feel overlooked, overpowered, or talked over by men, women in senior positions, or those who naturally tend toward greater assertiveness.

We might start off saying, "I'm sorry" or "This might be a stupid question, but…" when attempting to insert ourselves into a discussion, making a request that could be perceived as too direct, or feeling a diminished sense of power within an interaction or group. For example, when wanting to make a point or initiate a discussion, we might say, "Sorry to bother you," "Sorry, I don't understand what you mean," "Sorry, but would you mind…?," "I'm sorry to ask," and so forth.

What's next? "Sorry I exist"?!

This sort of self-silencing leads to feeling invisible, unworthy, powerless, and small. Ultimately, it can lead to a great deal of resentment and hurt. This pattern can send the unintended message that you really don't have much of a voice (because you've kept it hidden), or that you can be talked over and disregarded—and are okay with that (even though you're not). In time, you might have started to believe that staying in the background was acceptable to you, or perhaps it felt safer or even just familiar. It's interesting how we tend to create that which we actually fear and work hard to prevent, isn't it? This is how we become the ultimate silencer of ourselves.

DISQUALIFIERS: DON'T COUNT YOURSELF OUT!

Writer Tara Mohr (2014) discusses ways in which women minimize their impact with the use of qualifiers in their communications. Similar to "I'm sorry," one of these qualifiers is the word "just." Mohr explains that using this modifier—as in "I just want to add…" or "I just think…"—diminishes a woman's power. "Just" quickly disempowers what might otherwise be a stunning idea by connoting something more along the lines of "barely" or "I'm saying this with apology."

If you aren't confident about what you want to say or your right to say it, you might find yourself unconsciously falling into old habits that soften your impact instead of enhancing it. In an effort to communicate "I don't want to bother you," you might disqualify your statements by speaking quickly, using too many words, avoiding eye contact, or not using emphasis. The goal in these instances is to move toward using your voice based on the assumption that people will want to hear what you have to say. To do this requires slowing down, taking a deep breath, making a clear direct statement, and assuming your right to express your thoughts.

USE FEWER QUALIFIERS

Try reducing your apologies for making a request or taking up time. Observe your use of phrases that seem to act as disqualifiers or minimizers of your importance. Experiment with using fewer qualifiers.

Take out "just," "actually," and "sorry." Instead, try direct *I statements* and using "thank you" in place of "I'm sorry." For example:

- Instead of "I'd just like to add that I think…" try starting with your point by going straight to "I think…."

- Instead of "Actually, I'm not sure I agree here," try "I don't agree here. My impression is…"

- Instead of "If it's okay, I'd like to chime in here," try "I have something I'd like to add and haven't had the floor yet. My thought is…"

- Instead of "I'm sorry to take up your time," try "Thank you for making the time today."

- Instead of "Sorry to bother you," try "I have something to discuss with you. Do you have a few minutes either now or later in the day? Anytime between two and five is good for me."

LETTING YOUR BODY SPEAK

Your body language can have a powerful effect when it complements your voice and the message you are conveying. Social psychologist Amy Cuddy (2015) recommends expanding your body language to take up more space and convey a sense of being bigger, stronger, and prouder, as opposed to small, weak, and inferior. She recommends standing with your feet grounded and firmly planted, your head up, and your shoulders back with a straight spine. You can even put your hands on your hips like a superhero.

Similarly, if you are distracted, your body language will give you away. For instance, if you're having a hard time paying attention to the person you are speaking to, your eyes might dart around or you might turn your ears in the direction of other noises or conversations.

Take note of your body language in various environments, groups, and situations. What patterns do you notice? Check off those that apply:

☐ Am I crossing my arms across my chest? Relax them at my sides.

☐ Am I looking down or away? Lift my chest and head.

☐ Am I making eye contact or averting a gaze? Try holding eye contact a moment longer.

☐ Am I shrinking and curling my shoulders in? Open my chest and sit up straight.

☐ What unintended messages is my body language sending? Make a small adjustment.

SOFT POWER: USING MINIMAL ENCOURAGERS

You don't need to strike a power pose, hands on hips with your hero cape a wavin', for every communication, however. Smooth and effective communication requires flexibility and adaptability. To be taken seriously while retaining a natural sensitivity and conveying a heartfelt softness, you want to adjust your behavior in each situation. Use your voice in a way that is both helpful in communicating to the other person and still authentic to who you are and what you need.

When listening to someone, you can use *minimal encouragers* to show that you care or empathize. Minimal encourages are brief cues that let the other person know that you are present with them. They encourage conversation to continue and maintain intimacy. You probably already use minimal encouragers: making eye contact, titling your head in interest, nodding, making a particular facial expression to match the conversation, or saying "Uh-huh, yes, sure" in a genuine tone. All of these small gestures communicate "I hear you and I am with you in this moment."

Minimal encourages are helpful when you fear getting lost in a conversation, as they can direct your focus to what the other person is saying without having to speak a lot. This can help you tune in to what the other person is saying and keep you on track. Minimal encouragers are big connectors; they're empowering for the person using them (the listener) and validating for the person receiving them (the speaker). When you can engage in active listening, you and your ADHD brain can stay grounded.

SAY WHAT YOU MEAN

When asked your opinion or preference, state it. Don't deflect or give up your power of discernment, which is a common practice for many women. For instance, instead of answering a query like, "Do you want to go out for Indian food?" with "It's up to you," practice a more assertive response. Check in with yourself for a moment and then communicate with clarity what your authentic self wants to say.

Practice pausing to ask yourself what you think or feel, and then try some of these phrases, without qualifications:

- I think…

- I prefer…

- I feel like…

- I believe…

- I like/dislike…

- I would enjoy…

- I know I don't want…

Play with adjusting your comments, making them shorter and more direct. State your truth directly in basic, simple terms. Although kindness and care in choosing your words is important, oftentimes we overcommunicate when a brief, to-the-point statement would not only suffice but also have more of an impact.

Especially for women with verbal impulsivity, it's important to remember that people don't have to get the entire backstory or justification. If you see eyes glaze over, maybe it's too much info at once. Break down what you have to say into smaller chunks—you'll have more than one opportunity to speak. Ahead of time, you can also try preprocessing with someone, taking a moment alone to talk to yourself, or writing down a few notes. Identify your main points and what you want both parties to take from the interaction; this will help with memory and clarity.

Once you actually start to talk to someone, you may find yourself thinking about many other tangential ideas that you want to string together. If these ideas are distracting you or you are concerned you won't be able to remember them when it is your turn to talk, you can scribble them down on a notepad so that you can connect them later.

Maintain eye contact and keep returning to the moment at hand when you get distracted by sights, sounds, your thoughts, or even the other person's expressions. It's always okay to ask someone to repeat something or ask for a moment to gather your thoughts before responding. You can also just express something like, "I find that I'm so stimulated by your exciting ideas that I'm jotting down notes so I can remember to go back to them later!" (Who wouldn't want a compliment like that?)

Find ways to practice speaking with a slightly stronger voice. You can do this by connecting to a place within yourself that knows what you want to express about who you are. Find grounding in this space and hold here for a moment longer than usual to experience what it's like for you to claim that right.

Become More Visible

So far in this chapter we have talked about maintaining our space and sharing the stage, as well as not wandering off or being pushed aside. We have talked about holding our space through less accommodation and making ourselves heard through our stronger voice. Now we turn to making ourselves more visible.

LIGHTING UP: SHOWING WHO YOU ARE

We don't always want to speak up. We won't always want to tell what we think or feel. That is fine and sometimes quite appropriate. Remember, though, we can always choose to let our personality emerge more, even when we say less. We can light up the space around us without revealing a thing, just by emerging from behind the veil to let our true and natural way of connecting shine through.

🪷 *Sari's Story:* Passing for Nice

Many years ago, before diagnosis and medication, I met my husband's relatives for the first time at a restaurant over dinner. A few days later, I asked my husband-to-be what they had said about me. The word they had used to describe me was "pleasant." Now, I'm a lot of things, but pleasant isn't usually the first one that people who know me well would use to describe me. Looking back, however, I saw that I had, in fact, tried my best to be "pleasant." I was flat, careful not to offend, careful to smile, nice, agreeable, and a good listener. I didn't reveal too much about me except basic facts.

I actually still find, many years later, despite years of medication and success talking in front of large groups of people with ADHD, that it is an ongoing struggle to open up and show my true personality with neurotypicals. However, I have learned that I don't need to reveal my difficulties, or give a speech on ADHD, or defend the whole tribe. I have settled on the goal and strategy to at least show more of my true ADHD personality. I can talk more or faster, smile, laugh, and engage. At least this way other people know I exist and know my personality, even if I don't overexplain everything about my struggles or ADHD.

"Pleasant" was a turning point. An ongoing lesson I still am practicing today is to not try to pass for "normal."

Discovery: Becoming Visible

How would you like to let others see you?

☐ Smiling

☐ Laughing and enjoying myself

☐ Being silly or quirky

☐ Sharing my opinions openly

☐ Feeling comfortable in my own brain and skin

☐ Acting naturally

☐ Other: _____

Opening Up: Letting People Connect

We often want to be visible from the inside out, to let people feel our deeper emotions and to know how we feel about them or about life. Tara Brach (2003) talks about the Buddhist concept of a "soft heart." Thinking about visibility as a softening in this way means thinking about welcoming people with whom you want to connect by letting down your defenses a bit.

Sometimes, defenses wall us off from people indiscriminately. We don't get hurt, but no one can come in or give us anything of themselves. This leaves us idle; we can't give back because we're behind a wall of a fortress.

When we open, we are more intimately visible. We can do this with anyone, from the food server to your friend having problems. Opening is a mental concept that only takes a minute and a slight shift in perspective. Take a breath and feel yourself softening, even if you don't know what to say. Show up as yourself, fully and naturally, when you'd like to be seen and characterized as caring.

Reflection: Opening Up

Is there some way for you to open up and show more of the real you without having to overexpose what you choose not to?

_____

_____

_____

_____

How can you open to let people in a little closer, particularly when you care but don't know how to show it?

_____

_____

_____

_____

Giving to Others: Make an Impact

Sometimes we feel better about "shining" when we realize it is not separate from our mission or desire to give to others. It is not selfish to take up more room. Instead, shining is about valuing who we are and what we have to give. When we think of it this way, we can see that, contrary to our potential fears, it is selfish to deprive other people of who we are or what we think, know, or bring to the world.

Reflection: **What You Offer**

Shining isn't selfish; instead, it is one way to impact others by being visible and present.

What is your desired impact on others? What would you like to offer?

_____

_____

_____

_____

What are others missing out on by not seeing and knowing you?

_____

_____

What do you do sometimes that makes you less visible?

_____

_____

_____

_____

With whom would you like to become more visible?

_____

_____

It may be easier to try becoming visible with new people who don't know you and therefore don't have built-in expectations. Go ahead; try a few more smiles at the barista or a few more sentences to the neighbor. Ask yourself what side of yourself, or your personality, or your warmth or humor you want them to see that you typically hide. Record your experience in a journal or voice memo so you can hold on to it.

ADHD-Friendly Chapter Takeaways

🪷 Becoming a bold neuro-diverse woman means learning to take, hold, and share center stage by opening more, by giving of yourself, and by letting your true personality shine in front of others.

🪷 You can enhance your presence and impact by shifting your verbal and nonverbal communication cues to be more direct and less apologetic. This practice helps you step more fully into the life you want to live and the values you want to live by.

CHAPTER 9

Keep It Real

Being Actively Authentic

Every time you make a choice that corresponds with an inner sense of assuredness, truthfulness, and authenticity, you move closer to yourself. The awesome part is that, when you are most aligned with your genuine, core self—which has separated from the shame and internalized messages you have received about ADHD—you generate the courage and sense of freedom that helps you traverse the path most fulfilling and purposeful for you.

Authenticity is important to this work because your journey toward a bold life as a woman with ADHD really, truly must be uniquely your own—which is why this entire chapter is dedicated to the theme of keeping it real with yourself. There is no one-size-fits-all treatment for ADHD, because there is no one-size-fits-all approach to living your most genuine life in your unique brain, body, and context!

When you keep it real with yourself, you end up stronger: more aligned with your needs, more pursuant of your desires, and more open in your relationships. This has the domino effect of empowering others to mirror your increasing sense of inner steadiness. Yes, you read that right: being more authentic can help make the world a better place! The journey toward your most deeply fulfilled and supported self as a woman with ADHD can bring out the best in those around you too. This is powerful stuff! It will help you gain a newfound sense of peace, strength, and courage to continue confronting your vulnerabilities and internalized messages of shame that have held you back for so long. To help you do just that, this chapter guides you through the stepwise practice we, the authors, have created for women with ADHD called *mindful authenticity*.

Mindful Authenticity

The term "mindful authenticity" was invented to mean an active practice in which we are aware of when we slip into hiding or reactivity. It also means that we are aware that we're acting from a shame-based feeling or ADHD autopilot. This awareness practice leads to an increase in authentic relating and behaving.

When we learn to maintain awareness of ourselves and our feelings of authenticity, we are able to increase choice and the empowerment that comes from this, creating a new sense of agency and effectiveness. In a psychological sense, a "sense of agency" is a sense of control, a feeling that we are capable of initiating and acting on our choices. For women with ADHD who have often spent years feeling inadequate, incapable, and incompetent, cultivating this sense of agency is powerful and necessary.

Living authentically with ADHD requires an intentional slowing down, something that is naturally difficult for the ADHD brain. If you have felt stuck because of this, it's not your fault, and there is something you can do about it! The active process of engaging in mindful authenticity is meant to help create the mental framework to put on the brakes and assess your experience so that you can make authentic choices.

For the sake of simplicity, it is easiest to think of the process of mindful authenticity as an act in two parts: noticing and choosing.

Noticing

The first step to engaging in mindful authenticity is, as with most things, pausing long enough to notice. When we allow ourselves the time and space to notice our internal experience, we have a much better chance at engaging life intentionally and acting in accordance with our mission, vision, and needs.

Noticing requires that we sit with our inner experience for a moment, especially when the uncomfortable stuff comes up. In these moments, we have a chance to hold our deepest discomfort and fears with compassion, care, and curiosity. This helps us stay away from habitual self-defeating behaviors such as hiding, pretending, retreating, reacting, or melting down—and it makes room for new choices.

This noticing process is best imagined as a body scan, in which you lightly and compassionately observe and label your internal experience and subsequent behaviors. This helps you create enough distance from your experience of an obstacle or ADHD moment to actually make an intentional choice. And making an intentional choice means you aren't being led by and from ADHD autopilot.

When going about this work of noticing, it is helpful to remember that emotions, and the thoughts that accompany them, are information. They exist for good reason and can cue you in to what you need and where your boundaries lie. Emotions will let you know when you feel most alive or most dampened and oppressed.

Women with ADHD are often emotionally sensitive and can be emotionally reactive. We are more prone to emotional dysregulation, or flooding, when the emotional brain becomes hijacked, making it hard to slow down and access clear thought. So that stress and emotionality you feel? It's real (Combs et al., 2015). But it is also a helpful guide to what you need and how you are living.

Taking note of your experience allows you to link particular feelings or reactions to the ways you are engaging with others. Pausing to notice also invites you to see whether you are honoring your relationship with yourself.

Noticing Signs of Inauthenticity

When you are in a situation where your authenticity seems to be diminishing, try asking yourself these questions:

- Am I experiencing a sudden drop in mood or sense of well-being?

- Am I embracing or resisting healthy vulnerability?

- Am I holding back or reacting from an emotional space that is not reflective of my authentic self?

- Am I finding myself avoiding expression because I anticipate conflict or a threat to connection?

- Do I anticipate being misunderstood, judged, or ignored?

- Do I feel as if I'm not completely present or able to be myself?

These are a few potential early indicators that you are experiencing, or at risk of experiencing, the beginning of inauthenticity. What follows is a more expansive list of possible changes in mood and behaviors that suggest the need to pause, reflect, and move into intentional action.

Discovery: Noticing Emotional Cues

Check off emotions that are accurate descriptors of your experiences of inauthenticity.

When I am being inauthentic, I feel...

☐ A sudden drop in my overall sense of well-being

☐ Increased anxiety, emotionality, or reactivity

☐ Misunderstood, judged, or shut down

☐ Invisible

☐ Afraid of being found out

☐ The ache of old wounds arising

☐ Defensive or protective

☐ Angry, frustrated, or annoyed

☐ Other: _____

Discovery: Noticing Physical Sensations

When I am being inauthentic, I notice...

☐ A pain or ache in my chest

☐ A lump in my throat

☐ Knots, butterflies, or swirling sensations in my stomach

☐ Tension in my body

☐ Clenched teeth

☐ Tears behind my eyes

☐ Increased heart rate

☐ A sense of walls or protectedness in my body

☐ A felt inclination to make myself smaller or bigger

☐ Other: _____

Discovery: Noticing Behavior Changes

When I'm being inauthentic, I tend to...

☐ Shrink back instead of moving toward people or experiences

☐ Withdraw instead of becoming more involved or engaged

☐ Hide instead of revealing or opening up

☐ Leave a situation when I'd rather stay

☐ Stay in a situation when I'd rather leave

☐ Treat myself and others in a way I don't feel good about, instead of acting with integrity and self-care

☐ Dismiss my own best interests, needs, and intentions, instead of asserting myself

☐ Other: _____

Noticing Signs of Authenticity

If authenticity has felt inaccessible to you in your life, you might not be as intimate with your internal experiences of acting in alignment with yourself.

The following list is meant to prompt you to reflect on what authenticity feels like for you. How do you know when you are actually engaging according to your truth, values, and authenticity? Check off any experiences that resonate when you notice yourself being most authentic.

Discovery: Noticing Emotional Cues

When I am being most authentic, I feel...

☐ Engaged

☐ Excited

☐ Seen, heard, or understood

☐ Respected

☐ Bold

☐ Fulfilled

☐ Peaceful, relieved, calm, free, or joyful

☐ Sure of myself

☐ A sense of alignment with my needs and values

☐ A comfortable sense of space and a pause before choosing an action

☐ Other: _____

Discovery: Noticing Physical Sensations

When I am most authentic, I notice...

☐ I have open body language

☐ I smile easily and naturally

☐ Relaxed muscles in my body

☐ A neutral or calm feeling in my stomach and chest

☐ Excited butterflies in my stomach

☐ A steady heart rate

☐ An excited increase in heart rate

☐ A sense of ease in movement and action

☐ Some tolerable nervousness related to doing things differently and opening up

☐ Other: _____

Discovery: Noticing Behavior Changes

When I am most authentic, I tend to...

☐ Speak up when I want to

☐ Share parts of myself or my opinions in a way that fits my needs and the situation

☐ Make choices that suit me

☐ Express myself in ways that are kind to myself and others

☐ Act in alignment with my values, needs, and desires

☐ Pause before acting or speaking

☐ Stretch myself a bit toward growth

☐ Act more silly, quirky, or goofy

☐ Come across as more confident and less concerned with others' perceptions

☐ Enjoy being around people more

☐ Other: _____

Reflection: Mindful Noticing

What is the most important or interesting takeaway from this exploration on noticing signs of mindful authenticity? Jot down some notes about things that you want to be sure to keep in mind for future application.

_____

_____

_____

_____

_____

_____

Reflection: Identifying Common Triggers to Inauthentic Action

Describe a situation in which you experienced an inauthentic moment. Where were you? Who was there? What happened?

_____

_____

_____

_____

Describe your internal experience at the moment when you moved closer to inauthenticity and away from yourself?

_____

_____

_____

_____

Were there particular people, nonverbal cues, words, behaviors, events, or environments that were particularly triggering? Be as descriptive as possible.

_____

_____

_____

_____

How might you have handled the situation differently to choose authenticity?

_____

_____

_____

_____

Reflection: **Remembering Experiences of Authentic Action**

Describe a situation in which you experienced an authentic moment. Where were you? Who was there? What happened?

_____

_____

_____

_____

Describe your internal experience at the moment when you moved closer to yourself and intentional, authentic action.

_____

_____

_____

_____

Were there particular people present, nonverbal cues, words, behaviors, events, or environments that were particularly freeing? Be as descriptive as possible.

_____

_____

_____

_____

Choosing

Living with ADHD can feel like staring at the most fantastic blueprints—but without the tools to build. The process of pausing to move into noticing creates a base from which to move into intentional action. We call this second phase of mindful authenticity "choosing." In any given situation, you have a choice to move closer to yourself or farther away, to step into authenticity or to stay within the safe confines of your protective responses.

The greatest power that we have is to be fully ourselves. The ultimate goal for you to move toward, and what you have been building up to during this process so far, is the radical idea that you, as a unique and whole woman with ADHD, can choose to be fully yourself!

Choosing to Reveal Yourself

One way to engage in mindful, authentic choosing is to find a small way to intentionally reveal more of yourself. When you can do so, you will feel engaged in relationships and the world in a meaningful way.

There are degrees of opening. There is active pretending and then there is quietly not opening. Doing a quick scan to notice your internal and external experiences more clearly will help clue you in to the direction of your potential choices. For instance, very often feelings of not being heard or seen will make you feel disconnected or vaguely uneasy.

THE THREE-STEP PROCESS OF INTENTIONAL REVEALING

Now you will try a simple three-step process that you can quickly use to check in with yourself at those moments when you feel your internal experience shift. This process involves:

1. Asking

2. Scanning

3. Choosing

1. Ask. First, in any particular situation, ask yourself, *What do I want people to know about me?* For example:

- I want people to know I am smart, creative, and original.

- I want them to see that funny side of me.

- I want them to know I care.

- I would like them to understand my thoughts and knowledge on a subject.

- I want them to know more about my challenges and what kind of support I need.

2. Scan. Next, do a quick authenticity scan and ask yourself: *Given what I said I want to reveal, is how I am behaving allowing others to see me at this moment?*

3. Choose. Finally, choose. Now that you know how to recognize signs of more or less authenticity in yourself, as well as how to open in a given situation, you can decide how much to open.

Reflection: The Three-Step Check-In

After you have read the description of the three-step process of intentional revealing, answer the following questions to practice applying this approach.

Name and describe a situation where you would like to apply this process.

_____

_____

_____

1. Ask: In the situation you identified, what do you want people to know about you?

_____

_____

2. Scan: In this scenario, imagine yourself doing a quick scan and asking yourself, *Are my words and actions aligned with how I want to be seen and known?*

_____

_____

3. Choose: Given what you would like people in this scenario to see or know about you, what behaviors or statements would you like to choose to reveal yourself more authentically?

_____

_____

Not Revealing: "I Choose Not To" Is Also a Powerful Stance

A second way to enact authentic action is to deliberately choose not to reveal yourself, or at least not all of yourself, to certain people or in certain situations. The important words here are *deliberately* and *choose*. Sometimes, choosing not to reveal yourself is the best course of action.

Your experience is your own to reveal and share as you see fit. If you do not feel emotionally safe, or if you sense the need to protect a part of yourself, take an extra moment to notice and understand your experience within the situation. Is there a real threat to your emotional safety or a tangible consequence of acting in a more revealing and open manner? Perhaps there are some things you feel comfortable asserting or sharing, and others you don't. Again, there are layers and levels of engagement, and the choice to open or protect is yours at any moment.

> *Sometimes choosing not to reveal yourself is the best course of action.*

Let's say that you have decided not to share some of your ideas or opinions with a particular group of people. You may say to yourself, *I don't care to share my ideas with this group. They are not people I believe will understand or appreciate my ideas. I still like them, and they are a group with whom I can share some laughs, but I choose not to divulge or explain some other ideas I have.*

The point is to be intentionally selective and to know with whom and why you want to share your diagnosis or differences. In the same way, it's okay for you to be a proud woman with ADHD and save your personal experience, out-of-the-box ideas, and unique viewpoints to share with people with whom you want to engage about particular topics.

🪷 *Sally's Story:* Engaging Without Revealing

Sixty-year-old Sally has a particular group of lifelong friends who are pretty different from her in many ways. The group continues to share very fond memories and a great deal of laughs together.

"They are the only ones who remember where I lived when I was growing up, knew my childhood dog, knew my parents, and remember that boy with the freckles in the summer of the sixth grade who liked me. I don't have to tell them about my challenges or my creative ideas, and I like that! It's not less authentic. I am fully engaged when I am with them. We laugh and enjoy each other without me needing to let them in on everything I think and feel at this point in my life! This realization has been very freeing and made my time with this group of friends even more special!"

Sally genuinely likes to share a particular part of herself with certain people, and she feels comfortable and safe being selective in that way. She chooses wisely here and gets great satisfaction from this choice. Sally found that letting go of the belief that she needed to share every part of herself in every relationship was freeing and created harmony within those connections. While we all need intimacy, we need it in different ways, with different people, in different contexts. It can be relieving to enjoy less intensity sometimes! Sally has found a satisfying balance grounded in intentional choice.

Depending on the situation, you may decide to push yourself a little more; you may want to share more of yourself and shift the way you have been behaving. Perhaps now you are no longer afraid of being seen as different.

As long as relationships are healthy for you, they don't have to fulfill every one of your needs. Other people don't have to understand all parts of you. There are some friends with whom you may like to go to movies and others with whom you want to share your more intimate feelings. That's not hiding, that's choosing.

Pulling It Together

The following story encompasses claiming space, making yourself heard, and choosing to move toward revealing yourself and living authentically with another person. Cindy's story is a culmination of many concepts and practices discussed so far this in this book.

🪷 *Cindy's Story:* Taking Center Stage

Cindy, at forty-five, in addition to her chronic attention challenges, developed an autoimmune condition that required careful management.

Cindy had become increasingly challenged by the active vacations she and her husband had always enjoyed. For the past few years, Cindy would say yes to vacation plans but be in pain or not participate. Instead of telling her husband about the situation, she began canceling plans at the last minute.

Cindy was feeling increasingly bad about herself, her husband, their marriage, and these vacations! Her husband was increasingly upset about her inexplicable sudden cancellations. Though he understood and felt compassion for her pain, he had no idea what she was experiencing inside. He didn't have a chance to adjust his thinking or responses. Cindy didn't want to ruin his fun, but she actually wound up creating what she was trying to prevent.

The truth is, there were many things Cindy was interested in and still able to do with her husband. Cindy needed to find a new way that she and her husband could enjoy things—a way that worked for both of them, a way that wasn't worse, just different. With the support of her counselor and support group, Cindy discovered several new options she felt excited about. She settled on a cruise with different levels of excursions and a variety of activities.

At first, when Cindy quietly mentioned the cruise, her husband barely responded, "That sounds nice." She realized that she had to claim more time and attention if they were to get to a shared understanding of the situation and make adjustments.

Cindy did an authenticity scan and asked herself:

- *Am I shutting down to be low maintenance or no trouble?*

- *What do I want to say?*

- *What do I want to have happen?*

- *What do I want him to understand?*

Cindy tried again. Learning to quickly scan her internal reactions helped her figure out when she was shutting down or pretending. She noticed feelings of shrinking back, feeling let down, and feeling discouraged and disheartened. These all became shorthand messages to her to dig deeper and express more strongly, more directly, and with a fuller voice.

Next, she printed out the material and left it on the dining room table. She directed him to it when he sat down. He glanced at it and said, "That looks interesting." She went further and made a specific time and date to discuss the cruise. At this meeting, Cindy told him clearly and directly that she wanted to go on the cruise, explaining her rationale and what made this choice so important to her.

The space she claimed was, "Hey, here I am. I'm a woman with needs and desires, and I'm excited about this! Let's gear something around who I am, too, and what is compelling for me and authentic to me."

Center stage for Cindy! This kind of interaction actually improved rather than weakened her marriage. It made things clearer for her husband, who didn't know why she was messing up all their vacations at the last minute. It also gave Cindy the confidence to continue in this manner in other areas of her life.

This story shows how one woman learned to stop ignoring her feelings of acting in a way that hid her true desires and began to cause distress internally and in her marriage. She didn't have to make big shifts. There was not a big problem in her relationship. She just needed to be aware of when she was subtly backing off or backing away from stating what she needed clearly and repeatedly and finding a way to be heard.

ADHD-Friendly Takeaways

❧ Stepping into a bold life as a woman with ADHD will require you to practice being as authentic and aligned with yourself as possible. You can do so by practicing mindful authenticity and making intentional choices around revealing more about yourself.

❧ Mindful authenticity is a practice that will help you increasingly move to greater degrees of being more fully yourself with others. It requires pausing to notice what you are experiencing (such as with a body scan) and then deciding which actions most correspond with what you need in that moment.

❧ Intentional revealing is another way to practice moving into more authentic living and relating. There are three steps: ask, scan, and choose.

❧ With a bit of courage, patience, and practice, you can take practical, moment-to-moment steps to live into the radical idea that you, as a unique and whole woman with ADHD, can choose to be fully yourself!

CHAPTER 10

Create a *Real* Plan of Action

Integrating ADHD and Your Self-Concept into Your Unique Life

Look, we're keeping it real here. We don't have all the answers. *You* are the sole authority on your brain, your body, and your needs. Effective ADHD management is highly personalized. There is no right way to do ADHD. There is only *your* way.

We, the authors, want to help you create a support plan for ADHD. However, as part of our "radical" approach, and counter to traditional advice, we have found that strategies are most helpful when they *follow* rather than precede or substitute for the untangling process you have been engaged in. Simply put, you can't effectively maintain strategies when half of your mind is busy trying to manage your inner critic and oppressor. Now that you have gone through the process of untangling, you are more prepared to assert a new vision for your life, a new narrative about yourself, and a commitment to leading a bold and amply supported life as a woman with ADHD.

> *There is no right way to do ADHD. There is only your way.*

Traditionally, after medication, ADHD treatment focuses on the development of what are vaguely referred to as "strategies." Trying to follow these approaches, of which there are many, can be demoralizing if they are applied as if they are the way to "fix" yourself. There is no one size fits all when it comes to your unique brain and you as a unique individual.

The best approach is to get professional help and to *strategize your strategies*. Otherwise, you may conclude that you can't even do ADHD right! So, before we help you create an integrated ADHD support plan, we want to review some of the common "stuck points" that women encounter as they seek out support.

> **Strategize your strategies!**

How to Thrive with ADHD: Revisit This When You're Stuck

The work you have done throughout this book will give you the inner strength and boldness you need to look at ADHD support in a brand-new way: a way that works better, not harder. Once you have done the work of freeing yourself to live more fully, as a whole and valuable woman who has ADHD, you will find that you are able to think about your challenges, symptoms, and choices for support differently.

Assessing What Works

If you ask a woman with ADHD what she needs in terms of support, she is likely to reflexively respond with, "I don't know." This is especially true early on in the ADHD journey, but it can crop up at any time when there is a life transition or when the things that once worked suddenly fall short. Below are some considerations to guide you in those moments.

Reflection: When You Don't Know What Supports You Need

Recycle these questions! Before writing your responses, take a photo or make a copy of these questions to reread when you're struggling.

Which elements of your situation or struggle are ADHD related? Which aren't? It's not always an ADHD issue.

_____

_____

_____

What story do you have about seeking support or having ADHD challenges that might keep you stuck? How can you revise it?

_____

_____

_____

What are the tasks or situations that are certain to lead to overwhelm and shutting down? If you recognize your tipping points it will be easier to address them.

_____

_____

_____

Would it be helpful to reassess what you're doing for others and set new boundaries so that you can focus on your own needs right now?

_____

_____

_____

Where are you trying too hard, hiding your symptoms, or denying your needs? You can have needs and ask for support without disclosing more than you are comfortable with.

_____

_____

_____

What kinds of stimulation (or lack thereof) do you need to function optimally? There is often a fine line between too much and not enough stimulation. Find your balance.

_____

_____

_____

How can you make your peak periods of mental and physical energy work for you? Don't schedule or commit to mentally demanding tasks during your ADHD slump periods. It's a setup. Every time.

_____

_____

_____

Do you need tools (a reminder system), in-person or virtual support (a coworking buddy), a routine or strategy, or help brainstorming a plan of action? Maybe you don't need another organizing system; rather, perhaps you need a friend to chat with you while you put things away.

_____

_____

_____

What might you be avoiding in this moment? If you can identify what you're unwilling to experience, you can more easily lean into a small action step at a tolerable level of discomfort.

_____

_____

_____

Where is there room for compromise or small adjustments instead of big changes? Don't throw the baby out with the bathwater!

_____

_____

_____

What is your body telling you that you need? If you aren't hydrated, nourished, rested, or given hugs, your brain won't have the fuel to show up for you.

_____

_____

_____

What will make you feel most alive, centered, and capable? Choose that. Every time, every day.

_____

_____

_____

Check Your Lens

As women with ADHD, we have a tendency to describe the performance of neurotypicals in idealistic ways. We often compare ourselves to their level of functioning—one that is glorified and simply not sustainable for most people. Sound familiar? Embrace your neurodiversity!

Insider's Wisdom: **When Your Perspective Is Cloudy**

Here are some gems of wisdom we, and the women with whom we have worked, have found to be helpful when our view gets foggy and we need to regain our footing. In the space provided, add any other bits of ADHD wisdom that you find helpful, encouraging, or grounding.

- Define "good enough" and don't go beyond it.

- Just because it needs to be done doesn't mean you need to be the one to do it—certainly not all by yourself.

- You have ADHD. Let yourself have ADHD-related difficulties and needs.

- Aim for total imperfection!

- Be kind and remember, "Comparison is an act of violence against the self" (Vanzant 2013).

- Most people hide their struggles. Social media is one big highlight reel with no behind-the-scenes features.

- Someone else's success is not your failure.

- If you don't ask, the answer is always no.

- Write or doodle a design with your own mottos, quotes to live by, or inspirational words.

Get Creative

Women with ADHD notoriously have piles of magazines and books on the latest and greatest organization and productivity strategies, which present great ideas that are often ineffective for our unique brain-based challenges. Stop trying to fit into routines and strategies that aren't designed for your unique brain. Personalize your support systems, and make sure that you are using a particular method for the right reasons.

Insider's Wisdom: When Strategies Aren't Working

It can be frustrating when strategies that worked before aren't cutting it anymore, or they seem like the "right" tool to use but your ADHD brain doesn't seem to get on board. Here are some guidelines that might help you get unstuck when your strategies are failing you. (Remember, *you* aren't failing—the strategy is!)

- Notice when you keep expecting a strategy to work, even though it consistently falls short. This isn't your fault; it's not the right approach for you.

- Just because an organizational system looks pretty, or a particular strategy works for everyone else in the office, doesn't mean you should keep trying to make it work.

- You don't have to feel like doing something in order to do it. Remember our discussion of moving beyond your comfort zone from chapter 7? Find the edge where you can tolerate the discomfort of getting started or trying something new, and then choose one small action.

- Can you add movement, stimulation, or a reward to make the activity more engaging? Use the wave of more engaging activities to push you into less enjoyable tasks.

- Use natural mood boosters strategically. Tackle a hard task after a workout or a fun activity. Make boring phone calls from a beautiful park.

- Sometimes rest is the most productive thing to do. Take a break and then come up with a revised plan.

- Try, try, try again. You have the right to go on this journey imperfectly: to fall, get back up, and try something new or in a different way.

ADHD Support Essentials

While each person's treatment must be as unique as they are, there are some essential, fundamental components of ADHD support after diagnosis. Navigating through appointments, books, and support groups can be daunting, however, and it is easy to get overwhelmed and return to those old default positions and coping mechanisms. In this section, you will find information on the basic anchors of ADHD management, along with a guide to create your own integrated support plan.

See http://www.newharbinger.com/32617 for a list of recommended resources on ADHD support essentials. We have included a few favorites below.

Medication

The majority of people diagnosed with the neurobiological condition currently called ADHD benefit from medication, at least to some extent. While medication is not a cure-all and is not effective in every case, a consultation about psychiatric medication is a good idea after diagnosis. Drs. Hallowell and Ratey (1994) provide one of the most helpful explanations we've come across:

> The various medications we use in treatment of ADD can dramatically improve the quality of an individual's life. Just as a pair of glasses can help the nearsighted person focus, so can medication help the person with ADD see the world more clearly. (235)

We, the authors, believe the goal of medication for adults with ADHD is to make life easier for you. The intention is to not just perform better as judged by some external standard but to decrease distressing and impairing internal states caused by ADHD.

Depending on the resources available in your area, it is often best to work with a psychiatrist to help find the kind of medication (or combination of medications) and dose that will work for you and your unique brain. This process can take some time, trial and error, and patience. Remember, the goal is not to change you but to make it easier for you to be yourself and to feel well, with minimal side effects. It can be hard to find someone with knowledge of ADHD in adults, especially in women, so it is important to ask about a professional's experience in this.

Often, after a specialist and you have found a medication regimen that works, and if your situation is fairly straightforward, a general practitioner can take over the prescribing if that works better for you and if your doctors agree.

Remember that you are the expert on you. Don't be afraid to assert your needs, present your concerns, and ask questions. If the doctor gives several recommendations or instructions, consider making an audio recording on your phone or asking them to write it down for you. It's okay to get a second opinion, if needed. Bring your boldness and be your own advocate.

Environmental Adjustments

Sometimes simple adjustments to the environment or degree of stimulation can make a big difference in supporting ADHD symptoms. If the space isn't working, stop trying to make it work! While you can't always change your environment completely, there are often some small adjustments you can make to create a more ADHD-friendly setting.

Insider's Wisdom: When Your Space Needs an Adjustment

Here are a few ideas to get you thinking about how to make your environment work for your brain, so you can stop trying to make your brain fit into a setting that isn't ADHD-friendly.

- Consider the placement of your furniture; for example, some people work better facing away from a wall, and others need as little visual stimuli as possible.

- Ask someone else to be with you while you're tackling a task, even if they are simply nearby doing something else.

- Experiment with noise-canceling headphones and various forms of white noise.

- Adjust the lighting.

- Use a balance ball or disk on your chair to minimize fidgeting.

- Go to stimulating spaces where other people are behaving in ways that you would like to (a dance class, a meditation class, a coffee shop, a coworking space).

- Ask to have an additional panel put on your cubicle, or work from the conference room.

- Use visual cues in addition to auditory prompts.

Rebalancing

This is a tough one, especially for those who are natural caretakers, who have managed ADHD by putting out fires, or who tend to be overaccommodating. You have probably found that you need to frequently recalibrate your scales and that "balance" looks different depending on the ratio of stressors to resources at any given moment. It's not an exact science. Practicing mindful authenticity and intentional choosing are helpful in steadying yourself. Start by adding more of what feeds you. ADHD coach Regina Carey (2016) suggests, "Take a look at what fuels you and what drains you. Instead of giving a bit of yourself to everything, choose to feed your strengths and maintain your energy! Recognize the 'holes' in the fuel tank and fill them, instead, with things you love!"

Strategies

Remember how we, the authors, told you that this isn't a strategy book? It still isn't. There are already some great resources out there by our cherished colleagues, and we want you to soak up their wisdom too. See what they have to offer at http://www.newharbinger.com/32617.

To be clear, we aren't dismissing the importance of concrete tools, routines, and strategies in working with your ADHD brain. We're simply saying that they have to be personalized and come from a place of power, instead of pain, in order to be effective. Below you'll find some helpful basic principles to guide you.

Insider's Wisdom: **Basic Principles of Helpful Strategies**

Basically, most strategies have something to do with the following suggestions. Use these core principles as a foundation for how you approach your ADHD support plan, and individualize them to your needs and liking.

- Simplify. (Keep it simple, sparkles!)

- Use external prompts and cues. More than you think you need. (Perhaps way more?)

- Have more fun. (Definitely way more!)

- Assert yourself. Set healthy boundaries. Knowing "where to draw the line" (Katherine 2000) is an often undervalued and underused strategy. This means there's a solid market for boundary setting—and it's prime time to jump on in! (You'll thank yourself later!)

- Find your unique "attention patterns" so you know under which conditions your brain works best (Markel 2012). (Know thyself!)

- Balance the scale of stress to stimulation. (Yes, that means setting those boundaries. Eek.)

- Anticipate problems perceiving time accurately. (And maybe anticipate problems anticipating those problems, too!)

- Stay active and find ways to move your body that are fun and empowering. (Stop doing exercise you hate already! Stop that!)

- Connect with people who get it. (Yes, you'll be anxious at first. Leap!)

- Prioritize time in your zones of competence. (Boundaries, again. Ugh.)

- Nourish yourself well. Probably eat more protein and less sugar. (Sorry about that!)

- Find your motivators. (Playing with puppies, anyone?)

- Adjust your environment. (Have we mentioned that we love professional organizers? Twenty times? Okay, here's twenty-one.)

- Improve your sleep hygiene. Do whatever you have to do to make it happen; sleep disturbances are a problem for most with ADHD, and sleep deficits make symptoms worse. (Night owls, we're talking to you.)

- Go to the dentist! ADHD seems to be correlated with teeth grinding, which can get in the way of sound sleep. (Big smile!)

- Pause often. Choose intentionally. (Sounds so mindful, doesn't it? Hop on that bandwagon folks, it's not going anywhere!)

- Turn up the volume on your inner cheerleader. Don't believe everything you think. (Believe the cheerleader, though! She has a bullhorn.)

- You don't always have to be in the mood to do something. (It hurts, but it's true.)

- Keep your sense of humor! Laughing is a great mindfulness technique, and sharing that laughter with others is incredibly healing. In fact, there is an entire book of effective ADHD strategies for women that detoxifies shame with the laughter only shared stories can deliver (Matlen 2014). (Also, cat videos!)

Finding Help on a Budget

From late fees to copays, ADHD is expensive. Adults with ADHD are more likely than others to struggle with finances for a variety of reasons, including disorganization and trouble with money management, impulsive spending, forgotten bills and late fees, medication and doctor copays, and lower levels of professional advancement.

Insider's Wisdom: When You Are Worried About Finances

While a comprehensive review of managing mental health challenges and ADHD on a budget deserves its own book because it's truly a systemic problem, here are a few possibilities to consider when your finances are limited.

- Barter or trade services and goods.

- Visit virtual support resources (http://www.newharbinger.com/32617), from e-courses and webinars to productivity and support groups.

- Look for government and community programs that offer vocational training and other services.

- Start a skills-pool group in your community where people can trade and share services and strengths.

- Look online for drug manufacturers' coupons and other kinds of financial assistance. Ask your doctor for help applying.

- Ask professionals for payment plans and sliding scales.

- Search for supervised professionals in training to get costs down.

- Make use of community mental health centers. They often have someone available to help you apply for assistance programs, and many offer reduced rates or free services.

- Educate yourself on first-line, researched treatments. But beware of websites that proclaim to have the "latest and greatest cure." Be sure to carefully consider your options in treatment modalities.

- Share information you find with a provider. Look for a provider who is familiar with ADHD. Discuss the pros and cons to various treatment approaches that might be right for you based on your unique needs and history.

Assertive ADHD Communication Strategies for Women

Assertive and strengths-forward communication is one of the best ways to support your ADHD. Here are a few of our go-to communication strategies.

I Know I'm Messy, But What Are You?

Rather than an actual conversation starter, this question is one way to prompt yourself to prepare for communication by internally reclaiming your right to be on equal footing in relationships. In order to reclaim this equality internally, remind yourself that people without ADHD aren't perfect either, they're just imperfect in different ways. Mutual respect is what we are after. Shifting your inner perspective and using more compassionate or empowered self-talk can help communication about ADHD challenges come from a clear and empowered place.

Just the Facts, Ma'am

Describe your difficulties and what you need instead of (counterproductively) characterizing yourself negatively. If possible, suggest a solution, not just the problem, or ask how you might collaboratively brainstorm another option. For example:

- "I have difficulty remembering complex instructions by just listening. It would be helpful if I could write down what you're saying."

- "Can you email me those directions? I'd appreciate it!"

- "I'm most effective when I write out my thoughts before a meeting. Can you meet after lunch instead of first thing in the morning?"

Yes *And…*

Use "and" more often to bring the parts into a whole. This helps provide you and the listener with a more balanced, realistic, and integrated perspective. Try saying something along these lines:

- "I am competent *and* I have difficulty organizing."

- "I can do this part of the job *and* I will need some help in this other area."

- "I have challenges with organization *and* I am great at creating a warm, loving home."

If Flooded, Seek Higher Ground

When discussions become highly charged, it is normal for people to become "flooded" (Gottman and Silver 1988) by emotions and physiological reactions. In these instances, we feel intensely triggered, with all circuits firing, and we are physiologically unable to access higher reasoning. We can take a break and revisit the issue later when we are clearer, calmer, and more collected. While we feel the compulsion to "resolve" everything immediately, we will fare much better in those efforts once we've reached higher ground.

Support

Women with ADHD often talk about feeling needy or dependent when asking for help. This is certainly not the case; it is okay to have needs and express those within relationships. It is necessary, in fact, to be interdependent and lean on one another in healthy relationships. This is what gives us both roots and wings. Who would be happy to support you, if you'd only ask?

Professional supports that you might need at various points include assistants, coaches, organizers, bookkeepers, housekeepers, mothers' helpers, physicians, and, of course, therapists!

A big part of getting support may include working with a therapist. Asking for help is a bold move! There is a great deal of stigma out there about going to therapy. Most people enter the process with some degree of ambivalence and a decent amount of anxiety. However, good therapists provide a safe space to feel whatever you feel. Ultimately, the most healing element of therapy is the quality of the therapeutic relationship.

It is important to find a therapist who is knowledgeable about ADHD—or at least open to learning. Unfortunately, non-ADHD-friendly therapists have been known to misinterpret symptoms, like tardiness, as an indication of our underlying emotions about therapy. They may try to "fix" ADHD symptoms by making recommendations that feel dismissive ("Gee, why didn't I think of that?!"). This isn't our fault; these mistakes are made by well-intentioned, educated professionals who just haven't had much training or experience with ADHD.

If you really like your therapist but some of these obstacles arise, don't be afraid to speak to them directly about your concerns and how the interaction made you feel—as it probably elicited some degree of shame and frustration, reinforcing instead of healing old wounds. Asserting yourself and voicing your ADHD needs in this way can be very powerful and corrective.

Strengths

Your strengths are such an intimate and significant part of thriving with ADHD that we integrated a lot of information about identifying and optimizing your strengths throughout this book. Because our editor says we have a limited word count (a limit on words?! This is an ADHD nightmare!), please see our web companion for more resources: http://www.newharbinger.com/32617.

The following quote by Ellen Littman (2018), the writer of the foreword to this book, beautifully expresses our perspective on embracing your strengths.

We cannot direct the wind, but we can adjust our sails. Women with ADHD cannot change their brain wiring, but they can reframe their experiences through a different lens. They can learn to embrace their unique strengths and aptitudes, celebrate the creativity of non-linear thinking, establish new priorities based on self-acceptance, and find ADHD-friendly environments in which they can thrive.

The Integrated Woman with ADHD

Women who live fully and successfully with ADHD tend to approach their challenges from an empowered, proactive, and connected inner space. They do not have it all figured out; instead, they have learned to hold themselves in compassion and give themselves permission to try again when the going gets tough—as it inevitably will for all of us. To be a bold, integrated woman with ADHD means that you:

- Still struggle—and do so with self-compassion and radical acceptance

- Have a compassionate understanding of where your limiting beliefs come from and choose new narratives to live by

- Are guided by values instead of shame and fear

- Allow old stories and fears to visit but not stay

- Find and harness moments when there are openings to push the bounds of your comfort zone

- Claim your voice, space, and worth unapologetically

- Dare to keep dreaming and renewing your life, with ADHD in tow

- Actively seek support and commit to the hard work with a soft heart

- Refuse to be diminished by shaming messages—your own or from others—and believe that neurodiversity is not something to tolerate but something the world can benefit from

Brave, bright, bold women with ADHD live within connection and lift each other up because we know one thing for certain: You can't do ADHD all by yourself.

Reflection: Pulling the Pieces Together

In this closing exercise, we invite you to more fully absorb and integrate the new pieces of your story—past, present, and future—and answer the ongoing question: *How do I create a life that works for me?* This may require review of some of the earlier chapters. Take your time.

Write an untangling statement that completes this prompt: *This is how my brain-based challenges are separate from my view of who I am:*

_____

_____

_____

_____

_____

_____

Write a statement of you as a whole person, including your strengths, challenges, personal traits, and values.

_____

_____

_____

_____

Write down your mission statement.

_____

_____

_____

Write down you vision statement.

_____

_____

_____

Identify all of the rights you want to claim and expand.

_____

_____

_____

_____

Identify some new possibilities that you want to experiment with.

_____

_____

_____

_____

Determine how you want to experiment with a stronger voice.

_____

_____

_____

_____

Decide how you will monitor your level of authenticity.

_____

_____

_____

_____

Pinpoint the kinds of support you need for your ADHD challenges.

_____

_____

_____

_____

_____

_____

Determine whom you need to add to your treatment team.

_____

_____

Establish what you need to do to modify your environment.

_____

_____

_____

_____

Determine some first small steps that will take you to the edge of your comfort zone toward growth.

_____

_____

_____

_____

Identify the boundaries you need to set (and with whom) moving forward.

_____

_____

_____

_____

Remember This

We want this chapter to end with a very special takeaway. If you remember anything from this book, we hope it will be these few, simple, "radical" ideas. You may want to post this list where you can see it every day!

- *Instead of trying to fix yourself, you can simply learn to be yourself. You can be clearer and more confident about who you are even with or because of your unique wiring as a woman with ADHD. Above all, remember...*

- *ADHD is not a disease to be cured but a unique way of being in the world that requires an individualized, comprehensive approach to a complex but fulfilling life.*

A Closing Letter

Let's get real about ADHD life for a moment.

ADHD hurts in ways that are both hard to understand for people who don't live inside of it day in and day out, and often inexplicable for those who do. It can really get us down, and that's okay. The key is not to stay down but to learn how to step up out of that shame-filled space.

We hope that this book has helped you realize that you needn't make a den in the negative place or visit there too long anymore. You don't have to hang back, waiting for ADHD to go away. You don't have to hide yourself away. You don't have to overexert yourself and burn out in service of passing for neurotypical or making up for "deficiencies." You don't have to sacrifice pleasure or self-care because your ADHD symptoms flared up this week. You don't have to do it all alone.

A fulfilling life is the result of pursuing what truly, deeply lights you up inside. So here's the big idea: you don't need to fix yourself to start living, to feel good about yourself, and to show the world who you are. You have ADHD and you always will, which has to be okay—even if it doesn't always feel okay—because it simply is the reality of your life. It doesn't define you; it is simply a description of how your brain is wired.

Just as you must radically accept and acknowledge the basic facts of ADHD life, you also have a chance to choose to embrace a new perspective and some important facts that go with it, such as:

- ADHD struggles will continue to manifest in your life, and so will your strengths, character, and determination.

- Your brain requires more support and preventive care than those of others, which presents opportunities to invest energy and attention into caring for yourself the way you would care for others.

- You aren't neurotypical and never will be, because ADHD isn't curable. Still, you are the only you there is, with something unique to contribute to the world, no matter how large or small you think that something may be.

- You might need therapy and/or other kinds of professional help, and that provides you with a rare opportunity for personal exploration and the chance to destigmatize the process of embracing mental health needs for others.

- You may need medication, and that has nothing to do with who you are as a person.

- You will inevitably confront judgment and stigma, and this is a doorway to rediscovering yourself, reinventing your life, and helping others with ADHD do the same.

It might seem unfair, at first glance, that you got the ADHD end of the stick. Since we only get one shot at this life, you might feel worried that ADHD will get in the way of becoming the woman you know yourself to be on the inside, underneath it all. You might find yourself racing the clock, pushing yourself farther and faster, or, conversely, falling back and retreating into yourself and hoping tomorrow will be the day everything changes.

As you know, however, everybody's got some suffering, some more than others. Many have great success, some more than others. Since no one makes it out alive, and this fact is the great equalizer of all things, it is also true that no single life is inherently more valuable or worthy or special than another.

Just like those neurotypicals you probably compare yourself to, you are allowed to have worth, value, and joy just as you are, with all of your challenges and hang-ups and fears and strengths and passions and quirks. Even with the forgetfulness, tardiness, messiness, and emotional storms.

You have strengths that have gotten you this far, and you may have contributions you have yet to offer. You may have a unique way of perceiving the world that helps you notice connections in hidden places. You may have an ability to deeply understand others' experiences of difference or difficulty, and a persistent ambition to discover meaning and purpose in the face of adversity. You may have a capacity to model acceptance to your family and communities, and your spontaneous display of quirkiness can light up a room and give others the permission to be themselves too.

It's not fair to yourself or to others to hold yourself back from life when you have so much to contribute as a woman who thinks differently in the world.

You have a unique perspective; share it!

You have a need for mental health care; advocate for it!

You think outside the box; encourage it in others!

You have intensity; light your fire and spread the light!

Because ADHD requires doing life differently, it can be a pathway to transformation if you show up and gently but persistently push the limits of your comfort zone. You no longer have to be of service to the pain that has tangled you in untruths and tethered you to a smaller life. Every day is a chance to live into yourself and your bright, bold life a little bit more—and a little bit more after that.

Since there's no time like the present, you might as well start right where and as you are. It's the only version of you out there, after all. So stop waiting and go ahead: dive fully into your completely, utterly, wondrously imperfect ADHD life. We dare you to be proud of it.

With gratitude for the lessons and inspiration that women with ADHD give us daily, we the authors leave you with this quote by Rainer Maria Rilke (1934, 27):

Be patient toward all that is unsolved in your heart and try to love the questions themselves, like locked rooms and like books that are now written in a very foreign tongue. Do not now seek the answers, which cannot be given you because you would not be able to live them. And the point is, to live everything. Live the questions now. Perhaps you will then gradually, without noticing it, live along some distant day into the answer.

With all our warmest wishes,

Sari and Michelle

P.S.

We would love to hear from you! You can always write us at Solden, Frank, and Associates, P.O. Box 3320, Ann Arbor, Michigan, USA 48106. Or send us an email through our website, https://www.soldenfrank.com.

We also encourage you to visit http://www.newharbinger.com/32617 for our recommendations for all the great resources out there!

Acknowledgments

We want to thank our editors at New Harbinger, Elizabeth Hollis Hansen, Jennifer Holder, and Marisa Solís, for their wise and steady guidance in shepherding this project through from beginning to end. We want to thank Denise Brogdon, whom we could always rely on to sort through the most difficult non-ADHD-friendly details to come up with a solution! Thanks to Jeanne Bellew, a trusted editor, who helped us shape this proposal and plant the seeds that became this book.

Great thanks to Ellen Littman for her friendship as well as her contribution to the field of women with ADHD and for lending her important voice to this book. We are forever grateful to the ADDA family, especially Duane Gordon, David Giwerc, and Evelyn Polk-Green, for their friendship, ongoing mentorship, and encouragement, which helped support and shape our careers. We are thankful for the ongoing kindness and support of our local colleagues, Geraldine Markel, Wilma Fellman, and our whole Better Together Team, including Regina Carey, Susan Hunsberger, and Jen DiGregorio. We also want to give a shout-out to our physical therapist, Brad Skinner (yes, we both needed that as the book deadline approached!).

Sari

I especially want to thank my husband, Dean, for his constant and unwavering support throughout this project and throughout the years. Thanks to my daughter, Daria; son, Evan; Lucille Solden; and Erica, who supported me during difficult times. I want to acknowledge a few of the many who supported me professionally at the beginning and throughout the years: thanks to Thomas Brown, Arthur Robin, Ned Hallowell, John Ratey, Edna Copeland and Steve Copps, Thom Hartmann, Peggy Ramundo, and the late Kate Kelly.

I especially want to give thanks to Michelle Frank, who mysteriously appeared at the perfect moment in time to enrich my world, my work, and my life.

Michelle

Foremost, I would like to thank my mom, Mona; my dad, Walt; and my brother, Matthew, for whom there will never be enough words of gratitude. Your abiding belief in me has made all the difference, all along. Thank you to Phillip, the twist of fate that keeps me believing in the unimaginable, whose support and steadiness sustained me. Thank you to the Solden family, who changed my life in ways too profound to articulate. The ADDA Board of Directors, past and present, never cease to inspire me and make a world of difference without asking for anything in return. I want to acknowledge the hard work and courage of the clinicians and researchers who dared to speak to and study the experiences of women with ADHD long before it was a trending topic; I also want to acknowledge those who continue to break new ground. Thank you to the Brabbs family, who kept the laughter and snacks coming. Last but never least, I want to acknowledge the best dogs and writing companions ever, Penny and Snitch!

References

Armstrong, Thomas. 2010. *Neurodiversity: Discovering the Extraordinary Gifts of Autism, ADHD, Dyslexia, and Other Brain Differences.* 1st ed. Boston: Da Capo Lifelong Books.

Brach, Tara. 2003. *Radical Acceptance: Awakening the Love That Heals Fear and Shame.* London: Rider & Co.

Brown, Thomas E. 2005. *Attention Deficit Disorder: The Unfocused Mind in Children and Adults.* New Haven, CT: Yale University Press.

Brown, Thomas E. 2013. *A New Understanding of ADHD in Children and Adults.* New York: Routledge.

Carey, Regina. 2016. *Make a Splash! It's Time to Take Action on Your Life.* Ebookit.com.

Combs, Martha, Will Canu, Joshua Broman-Fulks, Courtney Rocheleau, and David Nieman. 2015. "Perceived Stress and ADHD Symptoms in Adults." *Journal of Attention Disorders* 19(5): 425–434.

Cuddy, Amy. 2015. *Presence: Bringing Your Boldest Self to Your Biggest Challenges.* Boston: Little, Brown and Company.

Eichenbaum, Luise, and Susie Orbach. 1989. *Between Women: Love, Envy and Competition in Women's Friendships.* London: Penguin Books.

Gilligan, Carol. 1993. *In a Different Voice: Psychological Theory and Women's Development.* Cambridge, MA: Harvard University Press.

Giwerc, David. 2011. *Permission to Proceed.* Springville, UT: Vervante.

Goleman, Daniel. 2012. "The Sweet Spot for Achievement: What's the Relationship Between Stress and Performance?" *The Brain and Emotional Intelligence.* https://www.psychologytoday.com/us/blog/the-brain-and-emotional-intelligence/201203/the-sweet-spot-achievement.

Gottman, John, and Nan Silver. 1988. *The Seven Principles for Making Marriage Work: A Practical Guide from the Country's Foremost Relationship Expert.* New York: Three Rivers Press.

Hallowell, Edward, and John Ratey. 1994. *Driven to Distraction: Recognizing and Coping with Attention Deficit Disorder from Childhood Through Adulthood.* New York: Pantheon Books.

Hallowell, Edward, and William Dodson. 2018. "From Shame and Stigma to Pride and Truth: It's Time to Celebrate ADHD Differences." ADHD Expert Webinars, *ADDitude Magazine.* https://www.additudemag.com/webinar/adhd-stigma-accept-yourself.

Hayes, Steven, Kirk Strosahl, and Kelly Wilson. 2016. *Acceptance and Commitment Therapy: The Process and Practice of Mindful Change.* 2nd ed. New York: The Guilford Press.

Hinshaw, Stephen. 2018. "Girls and Women with ADHD: Unique Risks, Crippling Stigma." ADHD Expert Webinars, *ADDitude Magazine*. https://www.additudemag.com/webinar/adhd-in-girls-women-risks-stigma/

Katherine, Anne. 2000. *Where to Draw the Line: How to Set Healthy Boundaries Every Day*. New York: Touchstone.

Kübler-Ross, Elisabeth. 1969. *On Death and Dying*. New York: The Macmillan Company.

Lerner, Harriet. 1989. *The Dance of Intimacy: A Woman's Guide to Courageous Acts of Change in Key Relationships*. New York: Harper Collins.

Littman, Ellen. 2018. "No More Suffering in Silence." *ADDitude* Spring 52–55.

Lorde, Audre. 1977. Speech. Lesbian and Literature Panel, Modern Language Association. Chicago, Illinois, December 28.

Markel, Geraldine. 2012. *Actions Against Distractions: Managing Your Scattered, Disorganized, and Forgetful Mind*. Ann Arbor, MI: Managing Your Mind, LLC.

Matlen, Terry. 2014. *The Queen of Distraction: How Women with ADHD Can Conquer Chaos, Find Focus, and Get More Done*. Oakland, CA: New Harbinger Publications.

Mitchell, John, Jessica Benson, Laura Knouse, Nathan Kimbrel, and Arthur Anastopoulos. 2013. "Are Negative Automatic Thoughts Associated with ADHD in Adulthood?" *Cognitive Therapy and Research* 37(4): 851–859.

Mohr, Tara. 2014. *Playing Big: Practical Wisdom for Women Who Want to Speak Up, Create and Lead*. New York: Avery.

Ochoa, James. 2016. *Focused Forward: Navigating the Storms of Adult ADHD*. Austin, TX: Empowering Minds Press.

Ramsay, J. R. 2017. "The Relevance of Cognitive Distortions in the Psychosocial Treatment of Adult ADHD." *Professional Psychology: Research and Practice* 48(1): 62–69.

Redmoon, Ambrose. 1991. "No Peaceful Warriors!" *Gnosis*. Fall.

Rilke, Rainer Maria. 1934. *Letters to a Young Poet*. New York: W.W. Norton & Co. Inc.

Rogers, Carl. 1961. *On Becoming a Person: A Therapist's View of Psychotherapy*. Boston: Houghton Mifflin.

Rucklidge, Julia, Deborah Brown, Susan Crawford, and Bonnie Kaplan. 2000. "Attributional Styles and Psychosocial Functioning of Adults with ADHD: Practice Issues and Gender Differences." *Journal of Clinical Psychology* 56: 711–722b.

Ryon, Holly, and Marci Gleason. 2014. "The Role of Locus of Control in Daily Life." *Personality and Social Psychology Bulletin* 40(1): 121–131.

Shaw, Phillip, Argyris Stringaris, Joel Nigg, and Ellen Leibenluft. 2014. "Emotion Dysregulation in Attention Deficit Hyperactivity Disorder." *American Journal of Psychiatry* 171: 276–293.

Solden, Sari. 2002. *Journeys Through ADDulthood*. New York: Walkerbooks.

Solden, Sari. 2005. *Women with Attention Deficit Disorder*. Revised ed. Ann Arbor, MI: Introspect Press.

Steinem, Gloria. 1970. "Living the Revolution." Speech. May 31.

Strayed, Cheryl. 2012. *Tiny Beautiful Things: Advice on Love and Life from Dear Sugar.* New York: Vintage.

Ulrich, Laurel Thatcher. 1976. "Vertuous Women Found: New England Ministerial Literature, 1668–1735." *American Quarterly* Spring 28(1): 20.

Vanzant, Iyanla. 2013. *Forgiveness: 21 Days to Forgive Everyone for Everything.* Carlsbad, CA: SmileyBooks.

Walsch, Neale Donald. 2012. Speech. June 8.

White, Alasdair. 2009. *From Comfort Zone to Performance Management: Understanding Development and Performance.* Hoeilaart, Belguim: White & MacLean Publishing.

White, Michael, and David Epston. 1990. *Narrative Means to Therapeutic Ends.* New York: W. W. Norton & Co. Inc.

Williamson, Marianne. 1996. *A Return to Love: Reflections on the Principles of a Course in Miracles.* San Francisco: HarperOne.

Psychotherapist **Sari Solden, MS**, has counseled adults with attention deficit/hyperactivity disorder (ADHD) for thirty years. She is author of the pioneering books, *Women with Attention Deficit Disorder* and *Journeys Through ADDulthood*, as well as a prominent keynote speaker at national and international conferences. She serves on the professional advisory board of the Attention Deficit Disorder Association (ADDA), and is a past recipient of their award for outstanding service by a helping professional. Solden's areas of specialization include women's issues, inattentive ADHD, and the emotional consequences and healing process for adults who grew up with undiagnosed ADHD.

Michelle Frank, PsyD, is a well-regarded clinical psychologist who specializes in the diagnosis, treatment, education, and empowerment of individuals with ADHD. She draws from cognitive behavioral therapy (CBT), mindfulness-based practices, and psychoeducational approaches based in the latest research to help individuals with ADHD live fulfilling, empowered lives. Frank serves on the board of ADDA, the only nonprofit organization solely dedicated to helping adults with ADHD. She speaks nationally on issues related to ADHD, neurodiversity, and women's empowerment.

Foreword writer **Ellen Littman, PhD**, is a clinical psychologist who has devoted herself to the field of attentional issues for almost thirty years. In her private practice just north of New York City, NY, she focuses on a high-IQ adult and adolescent population, with expertise in identifying complex presentations of ADHD that may be overlooked. She is coauthor of *Understanding Girls with ADHD*.

MORE BOOKS *from*
NEW HARBINGER PUBLICATIONS

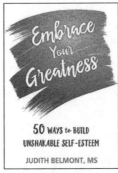
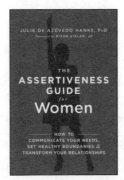
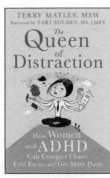
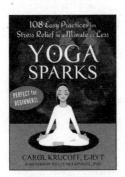
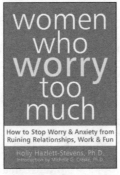
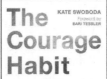
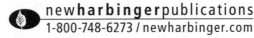

Real change *is* possible

For more than forty-five years, New Harbinger has published proven-effective self-help books and pioneering workbooks to help readers of all ages and backgrounds improve mental health and well-being, and achieve lasting personal growth. In addition, our spirituality books offer profound guidance for deepening awareness and cultivating healing, self-discovery, and fulfillment.

Founded by psychologist Matthew McKay and Patrick Fanning, New Harbinger is proud to be an independent, employee-owned company. Our books reflect our core values of integrity, innovation, commitment, sustainability, compassion, and trust. Written by leaders in the field and recommended by therapists worldwide, New Harbinger books are practical, accessible, and provide real tools for real change.

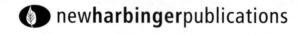 **newharbinger**publications

Register your **new harbinger** titles for additional benefits!

When you register your **new harbinger** title—purchased in any format, from any source—you get access to benefits like the following:

- Downloadable accessories like printable worksheets and extra content

- Instructional videos and audio files

- Information about updates, corrections, and new editions

Not every title has accessories, but we're adding new material all the time.

Access free accessories in 3 easy steps:

1. Sign in at NewHarbinger.com (or **register** to create an account).

2. Click on **register a book**. Search for your title and click the **register** button when it appears.

3. Click on the **book cover or title** to go to its details page. Click on **accessories** to view and access files.

That's all there is to it!

If you need help, visit:

NewHarbinger.com/accessories

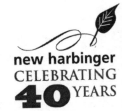

new harbinger
CELEBRATING
40 YEARS